The Here'sHealth Book of YOGA for all AGES

A completely fresh look at the health benefits that yoga has to offer, including advice on how to begin, warm-up exercises, breathing techniques, and how to build up your own yoga sequences.

Yoga transformed Cheryl Isaacson's life. It started an intense involvement in health and alternative medicine, which led to her joining *Here's Health*, Britain's leading holistic health magazine, in 1978. Previously she trained as a magazine journalist with D.C. Thomson's, writing and editing teenage problem pages.

Cheryl has studied yoga for twelve years, individually and with some of the country's leading teachers, as well as in India, Australia and the USA. In 1983 she qualified as a teacher of the Sivananda system and has also been influenced by the Iyengar method.

As main features writer for *Here's Health* she explored all the current holistic medical therapies and now, as a freelancer, contributes to other national magazines as well. She is also a student of graphology, swims, skis and has a profound interest in psychology and travel.

The Here'sHealth Book of
YOGA
for all
AGES

Cheryl Isaacson

THORSONS PUBLISHING GROUP

Wellingborough, Northamptonshire
Rochester, Vermont

First published 1986

British Library Cataloguing in Publication Data

Isaacson, Cheryl
  The Here's Health book of yoga for all ages.
  1. Yoga, Hatha
  I. Title
  613.7'046   RA781.7

  ISBN 0-7225-1210-4

Printed and bound in Italy

CONTENTS

Dedication: To my Mother

Acknowledgements and thanks to: Anne and
George Ivison and Anna Reid (for consultation and
rooms to write in), Mira Mehta of the London
Iyengar yoga centre (for invaluable assistance at
photo sessions), Harrods beauty salon (make-up at
photo sessions), Carita House (loan of leotards),
Michael Robeson and Lucie Joplin-Waters (cover
photo models) and, particularly, Simon Martin and
Leon Chaitow for persistent gentle encouragement.
All photographs by John Welburn, London.

Chapter 1

WHAT THIS BOOK IS ALL ABOUT

Why another book on yoga? Although there are many excellent books showing people twisting their limbs into intricate positions, it was felt that these did not always meet the needs of many who might benefit from simpler forms of yoga movement.

This book is about simple body movement, according to yoga traditions. By practising ways of moving, stretching and breathing which came into being thousands of years ago, it's possible to eradicate aches and pains, create suppleness and energy, and even delay signs of ageing. Yoga movements are also an excellent preventative measure. Even 10 minutes of stretching and breathing each day will increase life and energy flow to each part of the body, preventing the rigidity which leads to malfunction.

And the exciting thing is, everyone can do it. You don't have to be able to twist in all directions. You don't have to stand on your head. All you have to be able to do is move — in whatever capacity you, personally, can manage. Although the completed yoga positions may look complicated, and only for the young and supple, this book's aim is to show how simple stretches towards the finished posture can help you. And that includes everybody: the not-so-young, those who've never moved their bodies beyond the demands of everyday life, children and those people handicapped by a disablement which means they don't have full mobility. All these people can adopt a form of yoga to suit their own modern life in the Western world, and fit it into busy schedules so that in a short space of time they can improve their stamina, fitness, concentration and level of total health.

Yoga is not a competitive sport, or a fashionable challenging exercise. It's a way of doing things so that you are in charge, instead of being controlled by a wayward body that subjects you to its whims. It's a way of choosing how far you go, and when to stop. It's a way of getting in touch with yourself, discovering which parts of your body are truly alive and which are on their way to stiffening up and feeling dead. It's a way of introducing harmony between the myriad inter-connecting parts that go to make up you.

None of us is perfect. We all have our physical limitations and we are all, in some way, disabled. What yoga movement does is allow us to see more clearly what our personal possibilities are, and where our problem areas lie.

Yoga has been called a harmony between body and mind, and since the two are inextricably linked, it's not necessary to look far to see how one affects the other. The drooping, dejected body wracked by depression is an obvious example. But when you feel good, confident, fully alive and healthy, the whole stance of the body makes that clear. The energy system of body and mind is one and the same. And so, freeing the body from restrictions can help make the mind more clear, positive and active.

If exercise isn't really your 'thing', you'll probably be new to the indescribable sense of mind and body interconnecting to produce this clarity. Yoga isn't strictly exercise but it does have this capacity to get everything working in harmony. And the unique thing is, it won't exhaust or strain you like other physical movement. That's why it's especially suited to people who tend to avoid sport or anything that seems like sheer physical effort. You can get that 'high' without your body being in perfect shape and without endless training to stay in peak condition.

This yoga book is dedicated to those people who are unused to much bodywork. It's designed to help you get in touch with your body, to find out what you can do, to encourage you to action that's neither punishing nor tough. Of course, yoga can be both those, and a lot more, if that's what you want. But primarily, it can be valuable as the most gentle way of toning and tuning for everyone.

Yoga is a vast subject and there are many ways of going beyond its physical aspects and treating it as a spiritual path. Many books, and teachers, speak of its effect as a spiritual clearing house, enabling transcendence of the physical world and complete enlightenment. But it can be practised on many levels. In the West, nowadays, a harmoniously working body and mind are more immediately achievable through yoga than mystical experiences, and are perhaps more constructive if we are to withstand the barrage of stress that modern life gives us!

Yoga is very much a matter of personal experience, and how far you take the practice, and for what purpose, is up to you. The person ready for some sort of spiritual direction can find it through yoga. The person who is interested in improving his or her physical body will get that from yoga practice too. This book is aimed towards the latter, though don't be surprised if you get some unexpected results that aren't just physical too!

At this stage, I'm going to talk about my own experience of yoga. Each person who takes up the practice of yoga will have his or her story to tell, and all will be different, based on what their needs were, where and with whom they practised. But all will have some similarities, and that's what brings together a sort of yoga fraternity, so that wherever you go, yoga people seem to enjoy a common understanding.

At first my yoga practice was difficult. I had always avoided all sorts of exercise like the plague, and although I was in my early twenties when I went to my first yoga class, my body was very tense. Looking at the rest of the class — and the gorgeous, red-haired girl who demonstrated the postures — it seemed you had to be incredibly supple before you could do anything at all. Everybody seemed to move as if their joints had been freshly oiled! I was sure I'd never be able to get into any of the positions I saw them accomplish.

I was wrong. One thing you learn in yoga is never to look at what others are doing — and not to despair! It really doesn't matter what anyone else can do. What you are doing is just as good for you as any accomplished-looking posture is for someone else — and remember, they might have been doing yoga ten times longer than you. Yes, there are completed postures to aim at, but these are examples of perfection and few of us, let alone beginners, are able or expected to get into them. Whatever you can do to approximate towards them will stretch your own body, moving it in the right way — in your own way.

Gradually I grasped this fact. It took surprisingly little time for the initial stiffness to wear off, and for me to feel my postures were a bit more like those of the red-haired yoga model. I began to feel I was getting somewhere. That's part of the beauty of yoga. Improvements are not that hard to achieve — especially in the beginning. Whereas one week you can't get that right knee to reach anywhere near the floor, the next week,

miraculously, it's edged further towards it. It's neither miracle nor magic, of course. It's sheer regular and determined practice. But there's no force, no sense that 'I *must* get to that point'. If you practise, you get results. The body obeys, it works. Things start to happen.

To begin with there's increased flexibility. Along with this comes another discovery. Whereas before, you probably didn't notice your body that much, now you will be supremely aware of what's going on. It happens in a subtle way (or at least, it did to me). It's like becoming more aware of an energy system, a feeling within the body more than external changes. I began to notice how much energy certain parts of my body had, and whether everything was working in harmony or not. So there was a sense of co-ordination (when I was feeling at my best) — and mal-coordination, when something was awry. And, best of all, I began to see what I could do to *cause* this sense of togetherness, this flow of energy and vitality throughout my body.

I began to feel what co-ordination was really like. It must be the sense that athletes and dancers have, of being alive throughout your whole self. Mostly, we develop strength in some areas, those we use most — and often, too, strain and tension in these parts. Others are left behind. The body energy system becomes unbalanced. Your head and shoulders may be brimming with it. Your pelvic area, hips, thighs, might be sadly lacking!

All this doesn't seem to matter much as we go about our daily life. We manage, we get used to the way we are. Why bother to change? Because, when you start doing movements designed to work on the body *as a whole,* it feels a whole lot better! You find your overall energy improves, you feel clearer, sharper, more able in many directions. Usually it's the movements we like doing least that tell most about where we're going wrong. Some people find it excruciating to bend backwards, their spine seems to lock rigid. Usually these are the postures we pay least attention to, even in yoga classes. 'I can't do that one,' we say, giving up while congratulating ourselves on how far we can go in the posture we like because it feels comfortable.

But it's most important to learn from our difficulties. A hard backbend, a knee that won't bend at right angles, a locked shoulder, all need more attention than the things you can do readily. Concentrating your attention on just one section of the exercises will soon become self-limiting. You'll feel uncomfortable, your body will tell you there's something wrong. You'll start to work for more energy and life in areas of difficulty. That's how it was for me, and as I did so, my overall flexibility improved and one posture helped another, even those I thought I could do well.

Increased flexibility, I found, actually made my body stronger. Flexibility allows far more energy flow through a muscle, and thus you can work with it rather than it working against you. Unless you are strong throughout the whole body, it won't be possible to do certain postures — even those which don't seem to use your weaker areas. Thus a well-flexed and strengthened big toe will help you to stretch your upper body — because where would we be without the balance and support coming from our toes? That's the sort of thing you gradually come to recognize through yoga — you can be aware of your toes even when you're stretching your back!

For me, this sense of balance, of each part of the body working in harmony, of poise and lightness, gradually extended far beyond the yoga session. I felt much calmer after a class, and I wanted to work on my own to achieve that feeling. I soon found that a short session each morning set me up for the day. Without 10 or 15 minutes yoga stretching I was sluggish, feeling something was missing. It was almost like going out without brushing my teeth or washing properly. Something had been neglected, without which I wasn't quite fit to face the world.

Another thing I quickly felt, and wondered at, in my own yoga practice was its power to rejuvenate and relax. Often I'd go to my class at the end of the working day feeling very tired. It took all my effort to get there, and a physical work-out was the last thing I thought I needed. But slowly, even when I was feeling fit for nothing, the power started to work. The tiredness left, and replacing it was a renewed flow of energy. Often, the harder I worked, the better I felt. Somehow it wasn't like the physical effort spent in sport or other physical activity. It was a concentrated attention of everything in you, body and mind. It pulled the energy together again, from some deep inner source. It worked every time. The more tired I felt to begin with, the greater the benefit.

Relaxation sessions always come at the end of the yoga class and are a great thing to look forward to. It's always a relief when the instruction comes to put on something warm (because your body temperature drops when you're lying still) and get covered up ready for final relaxation, no matter how much you've enjoyed the class.

Sometimes you drop off, but that's not really the point. The aim in a relaxation session is to allow you to relax with conscious awareness. Then you can use the techniques to relax yourself anywhere, at any time, particularly during tense situations when you would otherwise feel out of control. Although it's nice to go to sleep, it's much better to maintain consciousness and feel a relaxed peacefulness with clarity of mind. Relaxation is the classic way to go into meditation, which is a forerunner to the deeper spiritual experiences some people get from yoga. Traditionally the physical postures are all performed for the sole purpose of allowing this relaxation into meditation.

For me, the sense of a calm, clear mind was one of the major benefits of yoga practice. It happened at the end of my first session, and was certainly the reason I kept going back for more. I felt untroubled, as if nothing could upset me, and I recognized how rare and valuable that feeling was in the modern world. At the same time I felt more in harmony and was able to slow down instead of letting all the thoughts in my mind have their way with me! I was aware for the first time of what was going on in my mind — so there was a sense of clarity and detachment. It wasn't unpleasant, just the opposite. I was beginning to watch how the way I moved my body and the thoughts I allowed to go round my head affected me.

One major recognition was how increasing responsibility over the body led to control of the mind. Often this mention of 'control' has unpleasant connotations, suggesting rigidity and the inability to be spontaneous and 'ourselves'. But this sort of control is something different. It really means awareness, being in command. An awareness of what we're doing, and consciously doing it better. There's nothing spontaneous about sitting with hunched up shoulders or a sagging stomach, or about allowing ourselves to be poisoned by negativity or anger. There *is* rigidity about recognizing these things then 'forcing' ourselves to stop doing them! Yoga is about the middle path. Coming to a deep awareness and understanding about ourselves, and allowing ourselves to change what we don't want. It's often a slow process, it doesn't happen in a day. But gradually everything works together. We begin to think about what we're doing with our muscles and limbs, and to put things right, to harmonize. Then something starts to work on our mental processes. The feeling that we are in control physically helps us recognize what we are doing in our minds. Just as we allow muscles to become fixed in certain positions, so we allow thoughts to stick in our minds. Doctors are only just finding out what yoga practitioners have known for years — that much disease is linked to states of mind. Rigidity and obstinacy may give rise to constipation. The inability to be loving can contribute to heart disease. Blocking emotional self-expression may lead to throat cancer. It's worth a thought — and worth taking charge of our thoughts as much as adjusting our physical weaknesses!

The highest level of mental and physical control through yoga practice has been seen in the East. In some dramatic experiments yoga practitioners have been buried alive yet been sufficiently in control of their breathing to do without oxygen for hours. Others have stopped their heart beat at will. All over the world, though, there have been examples of people reversing the progress of hitherto incurable disease through yoga practice.

But like me, most people will go into yoga purely because they want to feel better in a vague, indefinable way. And in small, gradual ways, they will begin to do so. Physically, I feel much stronger now, and am less susceptible to disease. Those winter-time epidemics leave me untouched and if some illness does take hold, it seems to disappear more quickly nowadays and not leave me so depleted — a cold is the short, sharp cleansing and energising process it's supposed to be!

Another noticeable change is in the way my body looks. 'You look more substantial, somehow,' was the remark of a friend who hadn't seen me for some time, after I'd been doing yoga regularly for a year or so. I knew what he meant. I hadn't put on weight. I hadn't developed enormous muscle power. It was just that I was firmer, with body weight more evenly distributed. I no longer looked fragile.

When I do yoga regularly, I'm more aware than through any other form of exercise, sport or activity exactly how the energy is flowing through my body. I become more sensitive yet also more relaxed. I feel calmer, saner, more able to manage my life. I'm stronger and clearer-headed, slowed down yet acute, flexible yet stable. It can't be bad!

So here's a book for anyone who, like me, just

needs to feel better, act more in harmony, and make more possible for themselves. The way to use this book is *not* to look at the colour pictures, say 'I can't do that' and put it away again. It's to start with the small illustrations, and to follow the instructions so you do just what you can do. Go only as far as the first picture if you like. Feel what that position does for you. Then go further if you feel you can. If not — that's all right, that's the finished posture as far as you're concerned. One day it will feel right to go further. Remember, the stretch you achieve is the one that's right for you, and the one that will work for you.

Beginners often question how long it takes to 'be able to do it'. But remember — you *are* doing it! As soon as you lift those arms into a position, you're doing your yoga. For some of you, the big pictures may be attainable straight away. For others, you'll stay at picture number one for ever. *It doesn't matter*. All yoga needs is concentration on what you're doing at any given moment, not longing for something you may be able to do in the future. So do your yoga, and be glad about it!

People often ask, too, about different methods of yoga. The postures in this book represent an eclectic range of yoga teaching from various schools, all of which have been valuable to me. Some people prefer to stay with one version of yoga, but this is very much a matter of personal preference. There are several schools in the West, and an even greater number of individual teachers, all with their own nuances and all with something to give. Recently, I have become increasingly interested in the Iyengar method, which is very precise and detailed. It was originated by an Indian, Mr B. K. S. Iyengar, who has himself practised the traditional postures for most of his life and has brought them to the West, in particular teaching some famous people in this country such as Yehudi Menuhin, the violinist. So the postures illustrated owe something to the Iyengar method, but must not be taken to be representative of it.

Altogether, they are my version, up to this time, of everything I've learned in yoga.

Happy yoga-ing!

Chapter 2

WHAT IS YOGA?

Fundamentally, yoga is a system of practices whose aim is physical, mental and spiritual discipline. By working along one or several of the yoga pathways, it is believed that unity with our spiritual self will be attained, and the unsatisfactory, dualistic existence where we feel separated from our 'true' being (the state in which most people live their lives) will be overcome. The word 'yoga' means unity and signifies the oneness which embraces light and dark, hot and cold, male and female, and all the other manifestations of duality which we experience in this world.

Because of this 'higher' purpose, many people are put off yoga because they feel it is some sort of religion, or at least, imposes religious beliefs on those who practise it. Nothing could be further from the truth. For one thing, yoga can be practised to any level you choose, and the spiritual aspects, although important in the overall philosophy of yoga, may play no part whatsoever if all you want is a slimmer waist or more stamina! It's very much up to you and what you want out of your practice is usually what you get.

Secondly, at its deeper level, yoga is more of a universal philosophy than a belief system. To some extent, of course, implicit in it are the beliefs of the East, and in particular of India where it originated. These speak of man's ultimate goal being to get off the wheel of life and death, implying an acceptance of reincarnation and the concept that the soul is on earth to learn certain lessons.

But there are many references which appeal to anyone, anywhere, of whatever persuasion. Yoga writings talk of the battle between the ego, or the lower consciousness, which is greedy and self-centred, and the higher self which links us with a greater good. In essence, the yoga teachings incorporate truths which are found in all great religions and philosophical systems.

Yoga is at the moment undergoing a form of transition. Once seen as decidedly foreign and suspect it is now becoming accepted in the West by all except the last bastions of religious orthodoxy. More and more people are incorporating its ideas into their own traditions, and seeing the similarities more than the differences. The possibility of practising a 'Christian yoga' has been expounded by one priest, Dr Dechanet, who explains:

> I know well enough that the exercises in this ancient discipline furthered the discovery and establishment in man of clearly defined tendencies: non-violence, truthfulness, chastity, poverty. But I did not know, though I felt instinctively, that carrying out these exercises would produce in me a real need of living the Sermon on the Mount, of understanding and of grasping the true dimensions of the Christian Beatitudes both on the level of world history and on that of the inner life. [1]

But even if philosophy and religion leave you cold, there is good reason to take note of the ancient yoga writings. They simply make good, common sense, especially in our troubled times. There are many pertinent images in the Indian philosophical texts such as the *Bhagavad Gita*, which form the basis of yoga: our thoughts, for instance, are likened to ripples on a calm lake, disturbing its clarity. How often have we felt like that, when in the grip of a perplexing problem causing an over-active brain, endless streams of thought and sleepless nights — knowing that all the time underneath, was an untroubled mind, if only we could find it!

Other references in yoga mention the human spirit bright and untroubled like a flame burning in an undisturbed place. Again, that seems a relevant image in a world where everything seems geared to attack our peace of mind and deplete our strength. By practising yoga, we are told we can encourage inner strength which withstands these external influences that throw us whichever way they choose.

Beginners are often confused because the yoga teachings seem to advocate a kind of detachment from ordinary life. By allowing the lamp of your spirit to burn as if untouched, by keeping your mind lake-calm and clear, it seems as if the practitioner of yoga is no longer affected by what is going on. To an extent, that's true. Does this mean, then, that you stand on your head amidst a family squabble, refusing to get involved, and wait there till it's over? Not at all. People who have been doing yoga for a number of years will tell you they feel just as involved with those around them, and with the joys and sufferings of life, but that their reactions are less emotional and, possibly, less self-destructive. They become deeply aware, but less disturbed — they can deal with it all without losing their inner calm. It's certainly detachment of a kind, but used positively rather than negatively 'cutting off' from your nearest and dearest.

How and when did this intricate yoga system all start? The science of yoga is believed to be over five thousand years old. Where it originally grew up is unknown. Although its beginnings are associated with Northern India, it may have been brought from further East and an Indian style imposed on it. Classic yoga postures can be seen in ancient Indian statues and carvings and the writings are intricately bound up with a form of Indian philosophy known as Vedanta.

But how, you might be thinking, can movements form part of a philosophy? Traditionally, yoga consists of several disciplines and can be practised through different means. The one we call 'yoga' in the West is mainly hatha yoga, which is one of many paths. It refers to the attainment of unity through physical posture, including the use of breathing techniques and cleansing processes. It deals therefore very much with the physical body, and is perhaps the form of yoga that is most easily understood and practised in the modern world.

In fact, it's hard to practise one form of yoga by itself. The more you become involved, the more you can relate other yoga paths to your life. As well as hatha yoga, other forms are:

Karma yoga — the yoga of practical work. Working in the yogic fashion means working without thinking of rewards for yourself, but offering up your work for the common good, without anxiety or desire. Mother Teresa, the nun who saves dying children in Calcutta, is one of the best-known examples of practising karma yoga.

Raja yoga — the yoga of the mind, where mastery is gained over negative states such as doubt, anger, fear, which prevent attainment of harmony. Raja yoga is very much connected with hatha yoga as both work on immediate physical and mental reactions.

Jnana yoga — the yoga of intellectual knowledge, leading to wisdom and understanding of infinite truth.

Bhakti yoga — the yoga of devotion. Those who live the life of religious mystics are said to be practising bhakti yoga, as are the great saints and religious teachers.

Laya yoga — a subtle form of yoga covering esoteric energy systems. These energies are connected with different areas of the physical body and each are representations of the universe, controlling different functions and with their own specific elements, moods and images. Balancing the interaction of all these energies is another way of attaining spiritual unity and harmony.

Mantra yoga — a way of attaining unity through sounds. The vibrational rates of different sounds all carry their own balancing function and thus affect us in various ways. Using them systematically, as in chanting, can cause dramatic results in our own energy system.

Tantra yoga — based round the principle of transmuting the physical into the divine. The body is put through various ritual practices, some of which might be very extreme and even orgiastic, in order to release the spirit within.

Kundalini yoga — entails practices designed to release a force which is believed to rest at the base of the spine. The 'kundalini' is referred to in yogic writings as a 'serpent power', or powerful energy, which can uncurl upwards through the spinal column until it is released in a mystical, spiritual experience. Considered highly dangerous to practise except under supervision!

All these different paths of yoga interact and overlap. It's not unusual to find that practising hatha yoga regularly makes you more aware of your daily work, so that you approach it with a different attitude, to take just one example. Or it may spread into your religious beliefs, so you become a more devoted Jew, Buddhist, or whatever. The intellectual, who collected facts merely for the sake of knowledge, may start recognizing universal truths and gaining insight, self-knowledge and balance as he learns — that's yoga too!

The hatha/raja yoga systems, which are the most closely interconnected, have their own special techniques, and these were outlined by a great sage of yoga, Patanjali, around the second century AD. Patanjali's yoga code is the basis of most 'yoga' as practised in the West today, and it is as follows:

1. *Yama* The 'do's of conduct in everyday life: non-violence, truth, honesty, abstinence, forgiveness,

endurance, compassion, sincerity, cleanliness and moderation.

2. *Niyama* Methods of individual discipline — purity, contentment, non-aquisitiveness, self-study and spiritual work.

3. *Asana* The name given to the postures of hatha yoga — literally meaning a firm seat, whereby the body is in proper working order and comfortable in one position for a long time. Thus, the body can ultimately become a vehicle for spiritual powers, instead of preventing progress by bothering its owner with physical distress. If a person is constantly troubled by physical ailments (says the yogic philosophy), he will remain a slave to his body and this preoccupation will prevent him attending to self development. Keeping still for long periods of time aids in stilling the mind as well as systematically balancing the physical energy flow.

4. *Pranayama* This simply means breath control. It involves regulating the in- and out-flow of the breath, with breath retention while the lungs are empty or full. There are numerous breathing practices based on varying rhythms in yoga, and their effects range from calming and relaxing, to stimulating and energizing the whole system.

5. *Pratyahara* This is the start of the more serious, spiritual goal of yoga. It means 'sense withdrawal' and implies the sort of detachment discussed earlier, where the yoga practitioner is no longer at the mercy of instant reactions to surrounding activities but can withstand them by inner calm and concentration.

6. *Dharana* Concentration, the next step towards the full meditative state. The ability to focus single-mindedly on one thing at a time develops self-direction and encourages the practitioner to remain unperturbed.

7. *Dhyana* Meditation: the meditative state is often considered an integral part of yoga and can certainly be attained as part of yoga practice. Sometimes it's enough to practise the postures in a highly concentrated frame of mind, to induce a form of meditation. Other times, you can enter meditation through a series of mental practices directed towards stilling the thought processes. During meditation there is a sense of the mind relaxing while the impact of everyday matters becomes less. There is a profound recognition of 'being here now' and completely integrated with oneself and one's surroundings, without any interference from thoughts of the past and anxieties about the future. There is great clarity and acute perception; often nagging problems are solved and there is a sense of freedom and of all being well, absolute, and right.

8. *Samadhi* The Samadhi state is one which most of us are unlikely to attain in this lifetime! It implies a state of absolute bliss, where the mind and senses are completely clear and liberation from the cycle of life and death is imminent.

These, then, are the classic 'steps' of yoga through which the practitioner can attain perfection. Traditional writings warn of many pitfalls along the way. In particular, the more advanced yogic practices may induce certain occult powers which should not be regarded as examples of personal spiritual progress or used for their own ends. It might sound far-fetched, but these powers are not all of the bed-of-nails or levitation variety. Many people who set about the perfectly innocent practice of yoga postures find their senses becoming more acute and 'strange' things begin happening. They might find they are becoming more telepathic, for example. They know who's on the ringing telephone before they pick it up. They sense a friend's in trouble and turn up on the doorstep just when help is most needed. They know what someone's going to say before they say it. It's as though the 'sixth sense' or intuitive faculty is becoming switched on, and a new sense of power experienced.

Sadly, it is possible to become side-tracked into all sorts of games with this kind of power. Yoga writings warn against them because, unless you're very careful and especially altruistic, they can end up being ego-trips, of the 'look what I can do' kind — and that's not part of yoga at all! On the other hand, if your yoga does make you more sensitive and intuitive, and you use this power in a positive way, so much the better!

Many people have found that yoga practice has enabled them to become dowsers (using the intuitive faculty to find answers to specific questions) or healers. It's heightened their awareness so they know what foods they need at a certain time, or which remedies to take for an illness. It's improved their concentration and their body functioning in numerous ways.

But how, you might be asking, does yoga actually work? Is there any down-to-earth, measurable, scientific proof of what it really does?

Yes, there is. Yoga grew out of an intuitive knowledge of what was good for the body, mind and spirit of a human being. The ancient sages experimented and found, by practical experience, what the postures, practices and ways of breathing did by result. Today, scientific measurement is verifying that they were right. Actual changes in heart rate, skin temperature, and brain patterns show that the ancient yoga practitioners knew what they were doing even if they couldn't explain how.

There are several major yoga research institutes throughout the world. In particular, the Lonavla Institute in India and the Himalaya Institute in America are showing that yoga has specific, beneficial effects on the whole human psyche. Here are some modern scientific findings:

— The lotus position affects *muscular efficiency*. Low-level exercise was performed more efficiently by a group practising the lotus position for 40 minutes daily for 6 months than by a group who did no exercise. Oxygen consumption during bicycle pedalling was used as the test. (D C Salgar, V S Bisen and M J Jinturkar, 'Effect of Padmasana — a yogic exercise — on muscular efficiency', *Indian Journal of Medical Research*, 63 (6): 68-72, June 1975.)

— A balanced system including postures, relaxation, breathing and internal cleansings lowers the incidence of *asthma* attacks. Out of a group of 104 patients on 4- and 6-week treatments, 76 per cent had no attacks during the treatment period and improvements were noted by laboratory and clinical tests (M V Bhole and P V Karambelkar, 'Effect of Yogic Treatment on Blood Picture in Asthma Patients', *Yoga-Mimamsa*, 14 (1 and 2); 1-6, April and July, 1971.)

— Yoga relaxation can help manage *hypertension*. A group of twenty patients in, on average, their late fifties, practised smooth yoga breathing, muscle relaxation and repetition of a word in time with inhalation and exhalation (mantra yoga). They also used biofeedback machinery to check their own ability to relax. All except one were taking drugs for the condition, which most had suffered for around seven years. Average value of mean blood pressure of 121 mm Hg decreased to 101 mm Hg and total drug requirement decreased by 41 per cent. Five patients stopped their drug treatment altogether. In a control group, who merely rested on a couch, there were no significant blood-pressure changes. (C H Patel, 'Yoga and Bio-Feedback in the Management of Hypertension', *Lancet*: 1053-1055, 10 November, 1973). Further studies by Dr Patel have consistently confirmed considerable blood-pressure decreases with yoga relaxation methods.

— *Red blood-cell counts* increase with hatha yoga practice. Six weeks of yoga practice showed an alteration in the hematocrit (the percentage of

blood volume consisting of red blood cells) from 45.9 per cent to 47.5 per cent. Groups doing another form of exercise had no significant hematocrit changes. (V H Dhanaraj, 'The Effects of yoga and the 5BX Fitness Plan on Selected Physiological Parameters', PhD dissertation, University of Alberta, 1974.)

— Yoga practice *lowers the heart rate* and thus increases its ability to adapt to strenuous activity. A group of subjects who undertook yoga practice for 6 months showed a lower heart rate during the postures than those who went straight into them with no previous training. (K S Gopal, V Anatharaman, S D Nishith and O P Bhatnagar, 'The Effect of Yogasanas on Muscular Tone and Cardio-Respiratory Adjustments', *Yoga Life*, 6 (5): 3-11, May, 1975.)

Yoga breathing practices have enabled adept practitioners to slow their heart rate sufficiently to survive in sealed underground pits for prolonged periods. Yogi Ramananda of Andhra took part in two experiments, one for 8 hours and the other for 10. On entry his heart rate was 85 beats per minute, decreasing after half an hour to 60-72. There were no heart abnormalities during the trial period. (B K Anand, G S Chhina, and B Singh, 'Studies on Shri Ramanand Yogi during his stay in an air-tight box', *Indian Journal of Medical Research*, 49 (1): 82-89, January 1961.)

— General yoga practice aids the function of the *parasympathetic nervous system,* part of the autonomic nervous system which enables the muscles and glands to work efficiently. An experimental group did 2 months' yoga training, including practising the Cobra, Half Locust, Bow, Shoulderstand, and Forward Bend. The autonomic balance score went from 64.64 to 78.07, in contrast to a control group — from 62.25 to 67.77. The increase was sustained even when yoga practice was discontinued. (M L Gharote, 'A Psychophysiological Study of the Effects of Short-term yogic training on the Adolescent High School Boys', *Yoga-Mimamsa*, 14 (1 and 2): 92-99, 1971.)[2]

There are many examples from all over the world of yoga being used as a positive physical therapy, and increasingly science is proving that it works. One patient says about her arthritis, 'My hands became so crippled I was unable to lift even a cup of tea. The doctors wanted to operate. There must be something about the movements in yoga that caused the swellings to break up and go away. At the end of 2 years I was mobile again.' Another patient, who also used the Iyengar system, this time on cervical spondylitis: 'My chronic trouble receded within an unexpected short time. Though middle-aged, I can now perform some of the difficult asanas with ease and comfort.'[3]

Similar stories are told about all manner of ills — multiple sclerosis, diabetes, migraine headaches, unspecific backache — being significantly eased with yoga therapy. The hows and whys are yet to be fully explained. We only know that the ancient knowledge of the East still applies today.

1. *Christian Yoga,* Dechanet.
2. Experiment data given in *Science Studies Yoga* by James Funderburk PhD, published by Himalayan International Institute of Yoga Science and Philosphy of USA.
3. *Body the Shrine Yoga Thy Light,* B K S Iyengar, published by BI Taraporewala for B K S Iyengar 60th birthday celebration committee, c/o Nanavati & Tijoriwala, 11 Homi Mody Street, Bombay 400 023.

Chapter 3

PRACTICAL QUESTIONS AND ANSWERS

There are several questions the would-be yoga practitioner needs answers to before starting. Here are some of them.

Can I do yoga at home, or should I go to a class?
You can do yoga at home, but the best way is to use a combination of home practice and a good class. The trouble with practising only at home is that you may get into bad habits with no one to correct you. Yoga demands very precise body use and it's easy to do the postures while maintaining your usual way of moving, which may be lop-sided, working one area more or less than others, and perpetuating the faults yoga should be correcting.

One way of working at home is to use a mirror. If you stand in your natural way in front of a mirror, you will see, on detailed examination, that you probably stand with one shoulder higher than the other, or in an otherwise haphazard way! The object of yoga practice is to balance yourself, and to use each part of the body systematically and symmetrically. It's often hard to get to that point — but it *is* the point! A good teacher will spot these imbalances and point them out to you; obviously it's much more difficult if you have to feel them for yourself.

Doing yoga at home, though, is certainly better than not doing it at all. It will help you get the feel of the postures, and give you a good stretch. Follow all the instructions very carefully, and use your body and its reactions as a guide to how far to take your practice.

How do I choose a yoga class?

It all depends on where you live, but you should make sure the teacher is qualified. There are some exceptions who have never gained a qualification, but are so steeped in the yoga tradition and teachings that they have a lot to give. However, it is best to protect yourself by making sure the teacher has been checked out and deemed fit to deal with a class.

There are several yoga qualifications, but the best ones, in Britain, are those given by the British Wheel of Yoga and the Iyengar Institute. These teachers will have studied and practised for some years. They are also the only two qualifications allowed by Evening Institutes. Of course, there is no guarantee that all qualified teachers will be to your liking, just as those who have studied in other ways, or gained no qualification at all, may have just what you need.

So the only real way is to go to a class and find out what it does for you. If you come out feeling refreshed, relaxed, and as if something's happened — then stay with it!

It often happens, too, that different teachers are right at different stages of your yoga practice. 'When the pupil is ready, the teacher appears,' is a yogic saying. It often seems to be true. Just when you've learned all you can from one person, for some reason you find yourself changing to another without having planned it that way. Part of the yoga philosophy is that we draw to ourselves, through our unconscious urges, the things we need for our development (and this was written about long before the concept of the conscious and unconscious minds!). Thus our yoga teachers reflect where we are and what our needs are!

How often should I practise yoga?

The more you do, the more you'll get out of it! Like any activity, as you practise, you feel more comfortable with it, and become more adept.

Once a day is ideal, but you must plan your programme to suit yourself. The great yoga masters spend 8 hours or more at their practice, but that hardly fits in with an office job! The main thing is, don't punish yourself. If you fall for yoga and decide it's the only thing you want to do, fine, set aside however many hours a day you fancy. For the rest of us, even 10 or 15 minutes a day will be enough — and be beneficial. It's certainly more realistic to set aside a certain amount of time you *know* you can manage rather than attempting the impossible and setting yourself up to fail. Convincing yourself yoga needs at least an hour a day — then finding you can't spare the time — is negative. Recognizing that 15 minutes practice will do you good — and actually managing to do it — is far more constructive.

If it's not possible to practise every day, you can still get something from yoga whenever you do it. A longer session once or twice a week, for example. Primarily, yoga should not become a 'must' or an 'ought to'. It should be something you desire, and look forward to, and enjoy, as a regular part of your health programme.

So what, you may be asking, about the yoga programme outlined in this book? It certainly takes more than 10 minutes. If your time's really limited, here's what to do: just the warm-up session; *or* warm-ups plus the Salute to the Sun; *or* the Salute to the Sun alone; *or* Cat and Salute to the Sun sequences; *or* warm-ups plus as many of your sequence postures as you can (making sure they counter-balance each other: for instance, if you bend your spine backwards, it is essential to perform a movement which bends it forwards again) *or* Cat and as many of the sequence postures as you can (with the above proviso); *or* Salute to the Sun with some postures from your sequence, in a balanced way.

Where should I practise?
In a quiet, clean room. Don't try to do your yoga in the living room with the television on and the kids doing their homework. It will be almost impossible to concentrate, and concentration is important in yoga. You do need to be selfish about it, to find your own, quiet space while you work alone or with a friend/friends. A group may inspire each other, but yoga practice is a matter of individual concentration.

Your room needs to be warm, because cold places encourage stiff muscles and you won't be able to move easily. Also, you will cool down easily in the lying down postures and when you relax, and you don't want to get chilled.

A non-slip surface is important. Deep-pile carpets are unsuitable because you won't be able to balance easily. Polished wood floors are ideal, but you will need a mat of some sort to lie on. You can buy specially designed ones, which are comfortable and non-slip. Thinly carpeted floors are also suitable.

Have as little in the room as possible to distract you, but you should aim for a pleasant atmosphere. Some people like to light a stick of incense before they practise to perfume the room gently. It's nice to have the room plain, uncluttered and tidy and to keep it specifically for yoga

practice if you can. Appropriate the box room if necessary, or convert the loft!

Traditionally, yoga practice took place out of doors, which was all very well in the heat of India, but is not so practical in this country. If you can find a secluded outdoor spot on a warm day, though, try it. Many people find yoga outdoors has a special quality and is very refreshing.

Is there any special time for a session?
Traditionally, too, yoga is practised in the early hours of the morning. I have a suspicion that this could be because it simply got too hot later than 5 a.m. in India to move at all! But this could be the excuse of the lazy. Certainly, the air is fresher at this time of day and doing yoga early in the morning leaves you feeling set up for whatever else the day may bring. It could start a whole new routine!

If you're not an early riser, though, use any time of the day, with one stipulation. Yoga should never be done after a heavy meal, and it's best not to eat anything at all for at least 2 hours before practising.

Do I need anything special for my practice?
You should make sure that in your yoga room are the following:
A chair, for practising the early steps of the Shoulderstand.
A small cushion, in case you need to support your buttocks in some postures.
A tie, belt or scarf, for practising the Forward Bend and the Cow pose.
A blanket or two, for folding as a support to the head in the Headstand and for covering yourself up in the final relaxation.
Socks and a jumper for covering up in relaxation.
A long mirror, for observing whether your body is symmetrical.

What shall I wear?
Anything that's comfortable and loose and enables complete freedom of movement. Leotards and footless tights are preferable for women, and natural fibres such as cotton are the best. Many people like track suits or loose floppy shirts and trousers, but these make it difficult to see what your body's really doing and how aligned you are (or aren't!). For men, shorts and a vest do well, or baggy pants. Always do your yoga in bare feet or you may slip.

Is there a yoga diet?
Yoga is often linked to a vegetarian diet. But there are no hard and fast rules, except that you use common sense and be guided by the inner

awareness that comes from all the yogic practices.

The earliest yoga writings from the East recommended a diet which included grains (wheat, rice, barley), fruit, vegetables and dairy produce (milk, butter), plus honey for sweetening. It is recommended that the yoga practitioner avoids spicy, acid and bitter foods, including onions and garlic, which were thought to over-stimulate the system.

The belief that yoga is linked to vegetarianism comes about because its principles condemn killing or harming, so traditionally yoga practitioners did not eat fish, meat, poultry or eggs. It seems that there is a natural progression through yoga practice to becoming a vegetarian, and that the more yoga you do, the less meat you want to eat. There is no ultimate explanation for this, and a particular diet should never become obligatory, but rather, moved towards gradually and naturally.

On a physical level, one explanation could be that yoga makes you more sensitive so you become aware of a natural need for cleansing foods like fruit and vegetables, thus more likely to follow a vegetarian diet. On a spiritual level, it's said that vegetarianism is conducive to higher spiritual awareness, though it's uncertain whether that's because of the increased degree of compassion in the practitioner to living things, or because the 'energy vibration' of animal foods is counter-active to the energy of higher consciousness. Probably it's a mixture of both!

Whatever the reason for the diet you choose, it is important to get a good balance for you, and to eat fresh, wholesome, wholefoods as much as possible. Yoga should induce a whole new awareness of your needs on this level as much as on any other.

Must I do anything in particular before I start?
There are various traditional yoga cleansing processes, which help prepare you for the physical postures. Some, like swallowing a length of cloth then regurgitating it, to cleanse the digestive system or pushing a string or wire up your nostrils and drawing it out through the throat and mouth, may not appeal! The following are more adaptable to everyday life in the West:
Scrape the tongue gently with the side of a metal spoon, to cleanse it daily.
A modified form of nasal cleansing may be practised by sniffing a quantity of luke-warm water, in which a little pure sea salt has been dissolved. An invalid feeding cup aids this procedure. Tip the water through the spout, into

one nostril, holding the head on one side. Sniff the water up and spit out. This may feel strange at first, and even hurt the sinuses if they tend to be congested, but is a wonderful cleansing for the nasal area in preparation for yoga breathing.
A clean colon is essential before starting yoga postures. A good, balanced, wholefood diet will ensure regular elimination. Constipation is nearly always due to wrong diet — over-eating refined foods and too much fat (which can also include too much dairy produce). Other factors involved may be emotional stress and 'holding on' psychologically to resentment, bitterness, anger, and so on. The yoga postures in themselves help regulate the system so sufferers may find their problem disappears with practice. Never take commercial laxatives, which become habit-forming and may cause your own system to cease to bother about functioning naturally. Even herbal laxatives can have this effect. Try to establish regular, normal function by adjusting the diet, an exercise programme (including other exercise such as walking, running or swimming, apart from yoga) and gaining psychological balance.

What should I bear in mind when doing the postures?
The most important points to bear in mind are:
Stretch but don't strain.
Yoga is about gentle releasing, not trying hard to reach a given position.
Relax your body in order to go further as you stretch.
Increasing tension will only make muscles seize up and may damage them.
Remember, yoga is a gradual re-education.
Focus internally on how your body is feeling in any position, rather than how you look and how far you can go. Sense what the posture is doing for you.
Try to locate areas of stiffness within the body, and also where you are more flexible, as you do each posture. Yoga is not a matter of whether you 'can' or 'can't' do a posture, but how your whole body is co-ordinating. Become aware of what every part of your body is doing, and involve it in the posture.
Trying to 'get there' is not yoga — it's cheating!
Try to concentrate fully on what you're doing all the time. If you are thinking about what you're going to have for dinner while you're doing the postures, you won't get so much out of your practice as if you gently bring your mind back

to where you are and what you're doing. That way, your session will become a practice in harmony and co-ordination — both raja and hatha yoga!

If at any time in your session you feel tired, rest on your back on the floor as explained in Yoga Relaxation (Chapter 8).

Should I challenge myself to greater efforts in yoga?

'Challenge' and 'effort' imply strain and tension, which have no part in yoga practice! You should certainly work hard in a yoga session, and break down barriers and resistance both in mind and body. But the trick is to distinguish between striving in a pressurized way for goal and achievement, and allowing yourself to let go in order to release and use energy for your own natural, individual progress.

How soon will I get results?

It depends on the individual. Most people feel *something* happening in just one session, whether it's a pleasant and deeper sense of relaxation, or a few aches and pains from unaccustomed stretching! Sometimes you will see rapid changes, in strength, energy and flexibility; at others, you may reach a plateau stage where nothing seems to be happening and you may even feel you're back where you started. Often, changes in the body structure may occur which make certain postures, which you always found easy, suddenly difficult. This simply means you are using your body in a different, and more correct, way and it's adjusting.

Generally, don't be surprised if you get very different 'results' from each session. You'll just become more aware of the ever-changing state of your body!

Will it hurt? And what shall I do if it does?

You may get some aches and pains just after a session, or anything up to 3 days afterwards. Normally these are the sort of pains you'd get after any exercise, and they should disappear quickly. As you get more used to practising, they should reduce in severity, although even regular intense yoga practitioners say the pain never disappears, it just changes!

You should learn to distinguish between pain that is 'good' and that which is not so good, however! If at any time in your practice you get a sharp pain, stop instantly and relax.

If you have any medical condition, ask your doctor or medical practitioner if it is safe for you to practise yoga, and discuss with him or her the postures you may possibly do. People with medical conditions should always seek a qualified teacher, and ask advice before joining a class. There is no reason for anyone with a disability *not* to do yoga, in fact it has benefited many of the disabled, including those in wheelchairs. But they obviously require special teaching, so do get specialist advice.

Chapter 4

WARMING AND LIMBERING — THE YOGA STRETCHES

Starting hatha yoga is, basically, starting to stretch — and learning to relax. So what's so great about stretching? Try it and see. Cats and dogs do it regularly — why shouldn't we?

Here's how to do the complete yoga stretch — it will be unlike any you've ever done before. Make it the first thing you do in the morning, do it any time in the day too, especially when you feel tired, drained or stressed. And, in particular, do it at the start of any yoga practice; it will loosen you and make your body ready and fit for the coming exercises.

First lie on the floor, flat on your back. Spread out, move about, feel the contact with the floor. Maybe you haven't done this for years — perhaps even since you were a child. Try to regain that child-like feeling, when you moved without tension or inhibition. Now start to stretch. Raise your hands beyond your head, wiggle your feet. Try to reduce that hollow space you'll feel between the back of your waist and the floor. Now think about the area round your middle, and concentrate on stretching out from here. Get the feeling that you are 'loosening' the sides of your body, then let the stretch come up through the sides to the shoulders and the elbows. Stretch out at the wrists, then the fingers — and don't forget, all the time the stretch is coming from your waist, from the centre of your body. Keep hold of that stretch through the upper body, let it extend downwards now, through thighs and knees, right down to ankles and toes. Keep pressing down with the back of the waist, towards the floor, keeping the stretch in every muscle. Then relax. Let your body flop. Let go of everything. Release every bit of tension.

Once you've got the sense of it, start again, feeling that stretch coming out from the centre of the body, involving every little muscle and particle of you. And next time you release the tension allow a fuller sense of 'letting go'.

Now try the standing stretch. It's quite similar to what you were doing lying on the floor, but it involves slightly more effort because you don't have so much support!

Start with your feet about 2 feet apart. Raise your arms above your head, making sure you aren't sticking your tummy out or hollowing the base of the spine in the back waist area. It helps if you can get a sense of widening the space between the hips, spreading and creating room all around your tummy, so concentrate on this first, and again, loosen the sides of the body.

This stretch begins with your feet. Concentrate on ankles and calves, feeling a comfortable tension from within, almost as if it's deep in your bones. Bring the stretch up through your hips and sides, keeping your feet solidly based on the floor without putting too much tension in them. Then stretch through the shoulders and arms, raising them above the head without pulling them up — rather, let the stretching come from legs, hips and waist. Stretching here will enable the shoulders to loosen and the arms to become more straight. If you concentrate on stretching out at the hips, in fact, the elbows will automatically straighten!

Don't forget hands and fingertips — they need a good stretch too! Interlinking fingers and turning palms upwards, giving them a little pull, will help loosen out the joints. All the time you're doing this stretch, try not to sag in the middle, and, most important, never pull the body into position. You should simply feel a balanced stretch of equal intensity throughout the body. Allow a second or two at full stretch, then bring the arms gently down and bend from the waist, flopping and releasing as in the lying stretch.

This sort of stretch may seem a little awkward and even uncomfortable to beginners, so expect to practise a little before really enjoying the feel of it. Most of us tend to over-use some parts of our body, leaving others 'dead'. Stretching like this is the first step to familiarizing yourself with which parts of you lack life and energy and which are looser and more flexible. You may for instance find it difficult to involve your legs in the stretch, while your shoulders ease up nicely. Gradually trying to involve the whole body in the *equilibrium* of this stretch is a vital preparation for your postures, because this is exactly what you're aiming for in those more complex positions.

Although these instructions may be lengthy for such a seemingly simple movement, it's important that you follow them to get the most out of the pre-posture stretch. Doing it a few times a day will make you more energetic and supple. And don't feel you have to hold the stretch for long. At first, just get into it as fully as you can, then release, as holding demands that bit more energy! As your energy levels increase, you'll be able to hold for longer. And don't forget to breathe! Some yoga practices demand breath retention, often on a held stretch. But when you're warming up, it's best to keep things simple and breathe normally and naturally. You may find it *unnatural* and slightly strained to breathe in the stretched position, in fact, but if you don't you could find yourself feeling dizzy or faint.

Once you've got into the way of a relaxed, easy, full stretch, you have the basis of all the yoga postures, so do familiarize your body with this sense of opening and releasing before you do anything else.

Warm-ups

After stretching, concentrate on warming-up specific parts of the body. This will ensure that everything is sufficiently limbered and no damage can occur when you go into stronger exercises.

Here is a systematic way of dealing with each of the major muscle groups and joints in turn. It's not as lengthy as it sounds. Once you are used to it, you can whizz through this in under 10 minutes. Remember always to keep within your own ability, and if any of the exercises here sound too strenuous (they shouldn't be unless you are very unfit or unused to movement), go only as far as you are able.

1. Toe raises
Standing with feet slightly apart, raise up on your toes five times with feet pointing straight ahead of you, five times with feet pointing out and five times with feet pointing inwards at each other.

2. Ankle circles
Standing on one leg, bend the knee of the other leg slightly to bring the foot off the ground and rotate the ankle five times clockwise, and five times anticlockwise. Repeat with the other foot.

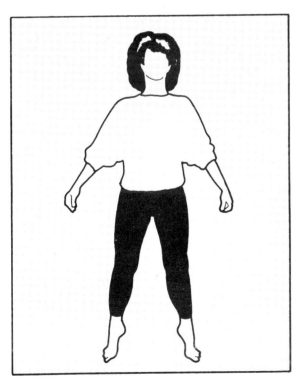

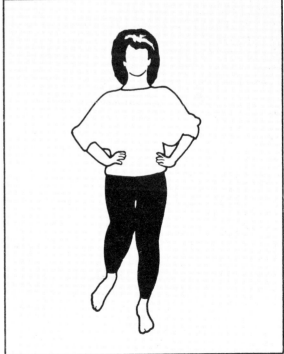

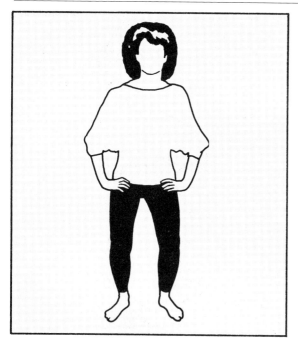

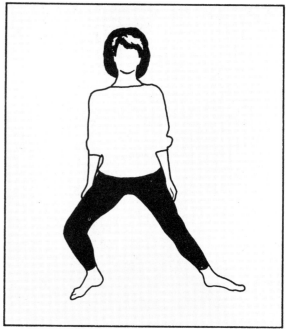

3. Knee bends
With both feet on the floor about a foot apart, bend the knees gently and straighten again, five times. If you have any trouble with knee joints, go carefully with this exercise.

4. Sideways knee bends
Omit this exercise if you have any knee joint trouble. With feet on the ground turned out at an angle, about four feet apart, bend each knee alternately, taking care that the upper part of the body remains straight. Arms should be hanging loosely. Do this five times each side.

5. Outstretched knee bends
Stand with feet apart at least 2 ft, with one foot completely outstretched to the side, at a right angle. The other foot should be turned in following the angle of the outstretched one but to a smaller degree. Turn your body so it faces to the side, in the direction of the outstretched foot. Place hands loosely on the thigh. Now bend the knee as far as you can — but you must keep the upper body straight and the other leg, stretched out behind, straight! Do this five times to each side.

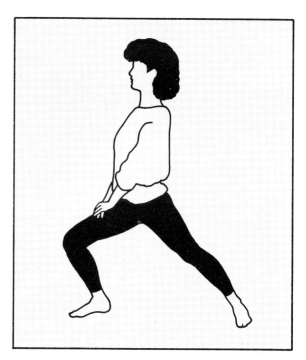

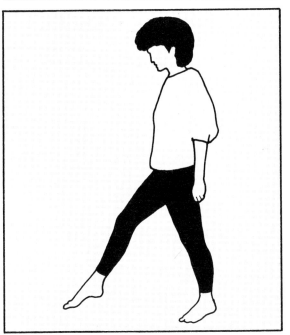

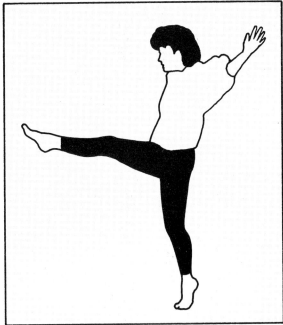

6. Leg kicks
Standing facing frontwards, kick the calf and foot out from the knee, making it as loose and relaxed as possible. Five times each.

7. High kicks
Take two strides forward to gather momentum, then do a 'high kick' — but remember to keep your back straight. You'll probably need to give a little jump or go up on tiptoe to do this — and concentrate on feeling loose in the waist. Repeat with the other leg.

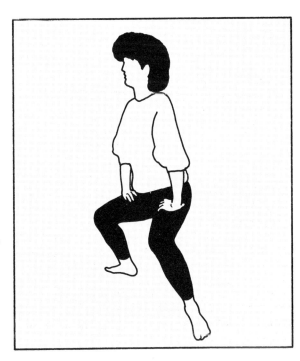

8. Squats
This exercise is not for the elderly or those who are unused to movement. Others should take it as far as they can — don't worry if that's not very far! With feet about 2 ft apart, facing outwards, and hands on the thighs, bend the knees, keeping the back straight. Try to keep this 'sitting' position for a count of five, without bending the top half of the body!

9. Hip circles

With feet about 2 ft apart, facing outwards, move hips forwards, then to the side, then back and to the other side. Gradually develop the four movements into one smooth circle, five times in one direction and five in the other. This exercise is not as easy as it sounds because it is almost impossible to do without moving the shoulders and upper body. The idea is to concentrate the movement in the pelvis, loosening the hips and waist. It's useful to look in the mirror to see what's really moving!

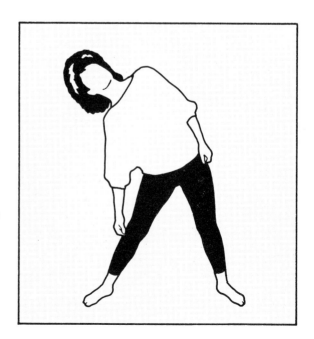

10. Sideways waist bends

With feet 2 ft apart, at angles, thrust one hip out and bend at the waist on the opposite side, with one arm hanging loosely on the bent side, the other resting against the body. It's important in this exercise to keep the head and upper part of the body in line on the same plane as the rest of you — as if you were 'sandwiched' between two boards! Both head and shoulders should be relaxed, with the head held loosely and naturally — mind you don't jerk the neck as you come up. Five times to each side alternately.

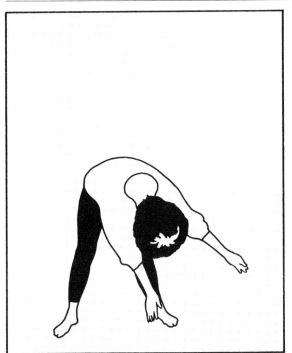

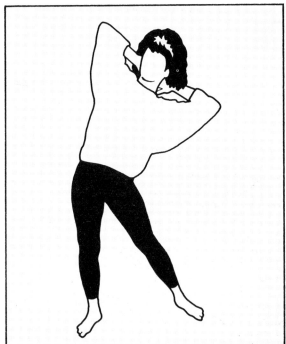

11. Circular swings
Do not do this exercise if you have high blood-pressure. With feet about 2 ft apart, bend at the waist allowing the head and shoulders to relax, and hands to reach as far down as you can comfortably manage. Gently swing round from the waist, so your hands move in a semi-circle from the front of one foot to the other, five times.

12. Waist circles
Clasp your hands behind your neck and stand with feet comfortably apart. Make big circles from the waist, dipping the head, coming up to the other side and bending towards the back. Five circles one way and five the other.

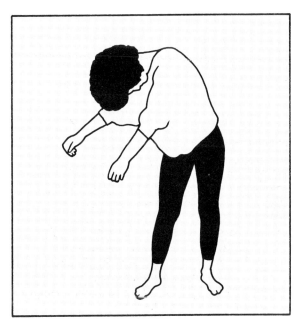

13. Waist swings
With feet comfortably a hip width apart, start by facing forwards then swing the upper part of the body from side to side from the waist. Arms should be hanging loosely at your sides and swing in time with the body's momentum. Keep the head lightly balanced, the feet firmly planted on the floor, legs straight and the waist, shoulders and face relaxed. Ten swings altogether (five to each side).

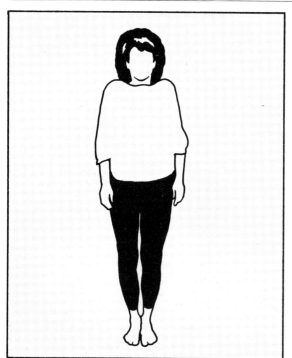

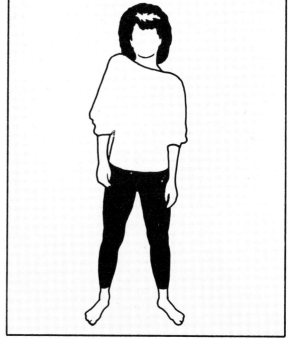

14. Shoulder hunches
Standing with feet together, raise the shoulders so they are as close to the ears as possible without tensing them. Make sure the head stays straight. Release and relax shoulders five times.

15. Shoulder circling
Standing comfortably, move one shoulder in large circles forwards, so it comes up close to the ear, five times. Do not tense the head or neck. Repeat movement in big circles backwards, then do the same thing with the other shoulder.

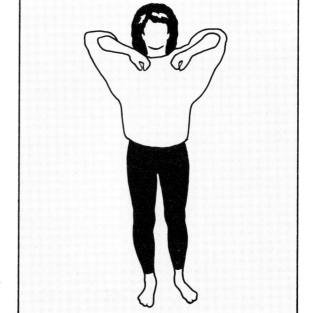

16. Shoulder blade movements
Work elbows round in big circles so shoulders come up and round as before, with shoulder blades moving towards each other at the back. Five times forwards, five times backwards. This exercise may cause a few 'ouches' the first time — shoulders are remarkably tense and this exercise is excellent for dispelling some of that tension, so persevere!

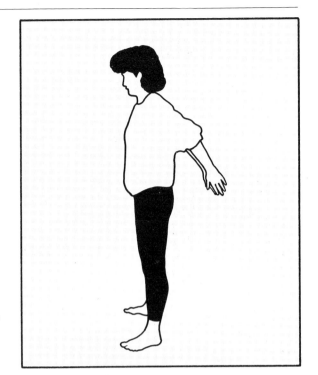

17. Arm swings
Standing with feet comfortably apart, swing arms up to the front then back down so backs of hands meet overhead and palms clasp together behind you. Keep the legs straight as a firm base and make sure not to tense neck or face. Five circles.

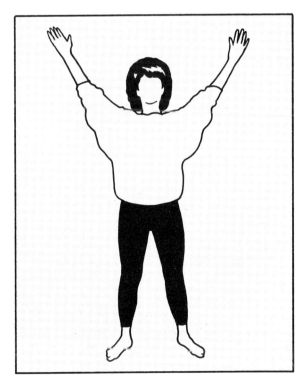

18 Windmills
Standing as before, raise arms overhead, brushing the ears, then bring them out wide to the sides and down. The movement in these arm exercises should come from the waist and the lower ribs, thus the rib cage is freed as well as the shoulder and arm muscles loosened. Five times.

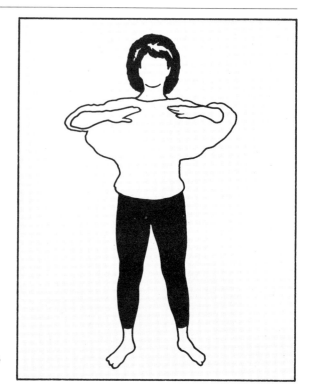

19. Chest flicks

Standing comfortably, bend elbows so fingertips meet in front of the chest. Flick elbows back and fling arms wide apart out to the sides, opening up the chest and rib cage. Five times — or even more, if you can!

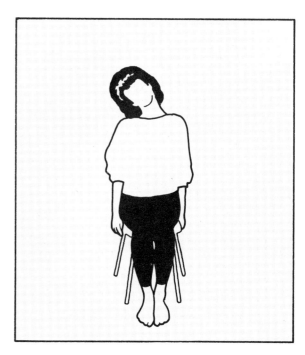

20. Neck bends

You can sit down for this exercise. Make sure the upper torso is firm and straight, and shoulders are relaxed. Very carefully, move the neck to one side, as if you were trying to get the ear to touch the shoulder. Please take care with this exercise and don't force anything! Raise the head gently and repeat to the other side. Five times to each side. You may get some small crunches and clicks, but the exercise should feel smooth and easy, and the neck will gradually loosen.

21. Neck rolls

Seated as before, with torso upright, head facing forward, dip the chin towards the chest then from this position roll the head very gently with ear towards shoulder, then dropping back, with the jaw dropping open, then round with the other ear to the shoulder and back to the front. Do this roll twice, then repeat in the other direction. It's important that the shoulders are kept relaxed throughout and the head should feel heavy and relaxed — keep control of it without holding it tensely. Again, you may experience crunches and clicks but please do not strain if you feel any immobility.

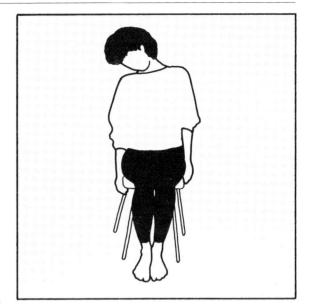

22. Face squashes

Tense up all the muscles in the face, screw up your mouth, nose, jaw, everywhere — make funny faces — then let go and relax! Repeat once more.

23. Eye circles

This exercise strengthens the eye muscles, which you are probably hardly aware of but which need their exercise and relaxation just as much as the rest of the body! Start by blinking a few times. Then look upwards, circle round to the 'three o'clock' position, round to 'six o'clock', to 'nine o'clock', and back upwards. Repeat, then do twice the other way round. Look forwards again and blink several times. Try to keep facial muscles as relaxed as possible during this exercise.

24. Eye diagonals

Look across to the 'ten thirty' position, then immediately across to the 'four thirty', up to 'one thirty' and back across to 'seven thirty'. Then up to 'ten thirty' once more. Look to the front and blink several times.

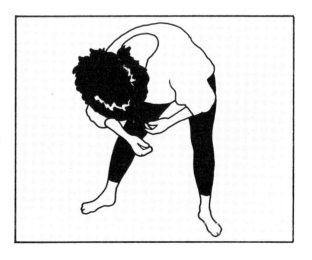

25. Shake-outs

Stand in a comfortable position, legs about 2 ft apart. Shake out the whole body loosely — first the arms, then fling legs out to the front, roll the head, allow everything to go loose and floppy and don't worry about how you look! Bend at the waist if you like, anything goes — imagine you're a rag doll with very little to support you. Then lie back on the floor and relax completely.

NOW you should feel looser, more awake, and ready to start some real work!

Standing up

Your yoga practice proper starts with standing up! But there's more to it than you think. And, as with many things, the simpler it sounds — the harder it is to do. Here's the yoga way to stand up straight: Check that the feet are together, the big toe and ankle joints just touching. Hands hang loosely at your sides, and you are looking directly ahead of you. It helps to check yourself in the mirror, or to have a friend look you over, because it is amazing how an unbalanced body may feel perfectly straight. And if you do find you're standing with one shoulder higher than the other, or one hip raised, don't worry, you're not a circus freak! No one is completely symmetrical — the way we were formed and the way we've used ourselves ever since ensures some imbalances. What yoga does is to make you aware of these and able to do something about them.

Once you have straightened your standing position, don't worry if it feels strange. You've probably been standing asymmetrically for so long, anything else seems unnatural. Gradually, though, you will get used to the 'right' feeling and your body will want to return to it.

Now feel your weight equally balanced on both feet, and distributed evenly on the whole of the underneath of each foot. Check where your balance usually lies — many of us 'dig our heels in', or teeter towards our toes! (See which part of your shoes wears down first!) Correct yourself gently, feeling your way into these slight posture changes. Then, without holding on to undue tension, but easily upright, imagine a plumb line holding you up from the middle of the crown of your head. The plumb line goes down through the centre of your torso, supporting and balancing you. Your shoulders are open and back — sense that you are gently allowing the opening to happen, rather than militaristically 'straightening up'. The back is neither hollow or sagging, the abdomen gently lifted, but again, not held tense. Allow it to take on its natural shape. Elbows and fingers are loose, hands heavy. Blink a few times to ensure the eyeballs are relaxed; drop the jaw and allow the mouth to open slightly and the tongue to rest behind the lower teeth. Come back to that plumb line; you now feel strong, supported and completely upright. Close the eyes for a few seconds and sense the balance and harmony of this position; once again, check for tensions that stop the energy freely flowing to all parts of the body, and allow yourself the freedom to stand, unhindered — enjoy it!

The stretching breath

Now you may start to co-ordinate breath and movement. From your balanced standing position, raise your hands upwards, bringing the palms to meet above your head. As you do this, take a breath in, allowing the inhalation to continue exactly the same amount of time as it takes your hands to meet. Take it slowly and steadily — the aim is a movement that does not rush at the start, nor speed up towards the end, but is controlled with exactly the same timing throughout.

Once the hands have met, your outbreath begins. Now you should gently lower the arms to your sides, with the movement lasting the exact extent of the breath. Hands reach the sides at the precise second the last bit of air is exhaled. It's not as simple as it sounds, because this exercise demands exact co-ordination and control — but practice does make perfect. When you think you've got it right — make it harder by going up on tiptoe on the inhalation. You may also stay in the arms-up position for an exhalation and an inhalation, before the exhalation down. Remember, everything under control, and both arms moving symmetrically! Done regularly, this simple exercise will bring increased balance and calmness.

Chapter 5

YOGA BREATHING

Surely breathing is just breathing: a simple, natural event. We do it without thinking, all our lives — and when we don't — that's the end! Can yoga breathing really be any different?

Yoga breathing still relies, like any other, on inhalation and exhalation. Where it differs, though, is in conscious use of the breathing apparatus — chiefly, lungs and rib cage — so that, instead of being a haphazard and often inefficient happening, breath is actually directed to a purpose.

Our breathing rhythms are intricately attuned to what's happening and how we're feeling. Most of us are familiar with the breath growing short whenever we're nervous or upset. Sometimes, when we're in a really anxious situation, it can be difficult to catch the breath at all and we may feel we're almost gasping for air.

Less easy to recognize is easy, relaxed breathing which most often happens when we're asleep. Notice how breathing deepens and becomes more regular as someone falls asleep, and note, too, how when all is well and you feel relaxed, your breathing falls into a slow, calm pattern. It's interesting, if you can, to watch how breathing patterns change during the day, according to our varied activities. Not just the obvious ones, like running upstairs or dashing for a bus, but situations like picking up the phone or dealing with a difficult neighbour may surprise us by their subtle influence! Often we may remain in a state of permanent 'arousal', as such tension is called, with attendant irregular breathing patterns, without realizing why we feel exhausted at the end of the day.

As you start to recognize that your activities, feelings and reactions influence your breathing pattern, it begins to make sense that working on your breathing can induce corresponding changes. Deliberately lengthening and deepening the breath when you're in a sticky situation won't make the problem go away, but it can help you to cope more calmly with it. Like the rest of your body, once you've taken charge of your breathing, you can use it in a positive way instead of letting it run away with you.

There are many special yogic breathing exercises which aim at specific results. Some may warm the body, others exhilarate; they may help you concentrate or simply relax. They may cleanse the system of waste material, improve organ function and induce meditative states. Yoga practitioners of ancient times knew thousands of ways to achieve health and happiness just by sitting quietly altering their breathing rhythms.

Today such techniques are taught only to advanced yoga students. Some degree of body control is a prerequisite for advanced breathing practices, for they are powerful enough to cause rapid changes which the practitioner must be able to deal with. But there is no reason why the beginning stages of breath control should not be learned by everyone. Most of us do not breathe nearly well enough, for all the same reasons as we misuse our bodies. Our functioning adapts to our needs — if we're office workers rather than long-distance swimmers, our lung capacity will reduce accordingly. We also tend to interrupt our natural way of moving, and breathing, with every trick imaginable. Physical and emotional inhibitions, ingrained since childhood; poor posture, learned or the result of bad furniture design; body 'armouring' out of fear and self-protection; polluted atmospheres — all cut us off from the easy, natural intake of oxygen which is our birthright.

We need to breathe as well as possible, not as well as is necessary just to keep us alive. For although we may not wish to cause dramatic changes with complex techniques, better breathing can help general health all the time. While we can live without food and even water for some time, as soon as we stop breathing, we die. The body depends on oxygen for transporting nutrients to each single cell, via the bloodstream, and also for oxidizing waste matter which can then be eliminated.

In the normal act of breathing, lungs are inflated between 16 and 18 times a minute. Their bellows-like motion is maintained by the action of both rib-cage and diaphragm, which are themselves driven by the nervous system through the respiratory centre in the brain. During inhalation, where the chest expands, the lungs are filled with air and its life-giving oxygen. When we exhale, the chest wall 'collapses' and gas containing stale carbon dioxide which has collected in the cells is emptied out. Breathing intimately affects the heart rate — if we hold the breath, for example, heart rate slows down. The most important chemical change is that whereas air when taken into the body contains about 20 per cent oxygen and 0.04 per cent carbon dioxide, expired air has in it only 16 per cent oxygen, and 4 per cent carbon dioxide. With each normal breath an adult male inhales and exhales around 500 cc of air. He has the capacity, however, to inhale and exhale another 1,500 cc, although even the fittest of us are unable to empty the lungs completely. The remaining 1000 cc — called 'residual air' — stays because of the lungs' 'dead end' shape.

Clearly, then, we could breathe much more efficiently. To do so would result not only in increased physical function, but more control over mental well-being too. Breath control in yogic terms is called 'pranayama', and inhaled air is said to contain a special force called 'prana'. This mystical prana is indefinable, scientifically unproven and nothing to do with elemental chemical construction. It is a basic principle of life and consciousness, as ultimately inexplicable as birth and death. As we inhale this force, say ancient teachings, we indeed become 'inspired' and renewed. Yogic writings, too, linked breath closely to the time of our life-span here on earth. Each one of us is born with a certain number of allotted breaths, they say. Use them slowly, and your life will be long!

So what, exactly, is the right way to breathe? As you read this and think about your breathing, most likely you will do some of the following: 'set' your shoulders back, throw out your chest, and/or have increased movement in the chest area. Many will remember the 'deep breathing' recommended as a child, when out on country walks — 'Breathe in the nice fresh air!' we were told, and sniffed appreciately in what we thought was the correct, deep, manner.

None of this, however, makes a lot of difference. Most common of all the inhibiting factors we impose on ourselves is a restriction in rib movement. To allow the soft, spongy lungs to expand thoroughly, the whole rib cage must move. Feel for yourself, as you read this, just what yours is doing. Breathe normally, placing the palms of your hands lightly on the upper part of the chest, just underneath the collar bone. Probably you will feel a fair bit of movement here, especially when concentrating on taking in as much as you can. Then place your hands over the lower part of the ribs. You can feel the curve of these divided sides of the rib cage just above the waist. Breathe exactly as you were, and note the difference. The movement will most likely be much less than the upper rib cage and some people may hardly feel anything happening here at all.

In fact, to breathe well, you need the whole rib cage working in unison, allowing the lungs to expand fully in order to take up oxygen. Likewise, a proper contraction of the ribs expels air from the lungs efficiently and gets rid of toxic waste. Many of us make the mistake of 'deep breathing' from the upper rib cage only, that is, we get an appreciable swing of the area immediately beneath the collar bone, leaving the middle rib section to its own devices and the lower ribs virtually rigid.

Another breathing fault is to get rib cage expansion and contraction the wrong way round. Yet, it can happen! Poor body use may have us expanding the ribs as we let go of air, and pulling them inwards as the breath comes in. Sit quietly becoming aware of your own breath and rib movements, and see if you're one of the many 'inverse breathers'. It's an easy habit to get into during childhood, but one which inhibits breathing considerably.

There are many other unconstructive habits (to call them 'bad' implies a measure of guilt — far easier on yourself just to notice what's there, then aim to change it!) such as full rib expansion on an inhalation, then leaving the ribs stuck out in mid-air, as it were, holding on to the inhaled air like you're never going to get any more! Or you may do the reverse — sending all the air out very efficiently, then 'sticking' at the point where you're afraid to let it all in again! Naturally, inhalation follows exhalation and so on, like waves on a shore — we should be neither holding back nor holding on. The body actually wants to be 'breathed' by the prana life-force; very often our fears and inhibitions don't let it happen.

No matter how much we've misused our breathing apparatus, it is possible to re-educate ourselves with fresh awareness. Basic, effective breathing techniques can be used all the time, and simple practices can help you keep calm or renew energy in specific situations. 'Deep' breathing is in itself rather a myth. More properly, we could talk about 'whole' breathing, and once you've recognized how to utilize the whole rib cage and lung capacity, you will feel more able to breathe freely and appropriately.

Yogic breathing practices are usually taught separately from the postures. This is because many are techniques in themselves, with specific effects as mentioned earlier, just like the postures. There are correct ways of breathing in the postures, but beginners should learn the movements thoroughly before attempting to incorporate breathing. Trying to co-ordinate breath and movement before you are ready may cause strain and confusion. In the posture sequences, it's best, then, to remember just to breathe freely and naturally as far as possible. Generally you should breathe out as you bend over or down into a posture, and breathe in to give yourself energy when lifting up out of a posture.

Now here are some very basic breathing exercises to do at home. I suggest that they could be slotted in after doing the warming and limbering stretches in Chapter 4. By that time you will probably need a rest period and focusing on your breathing will concentrate your energies in preparation for the postures, as well as making sure you are in the best physical state to begin them.

1. Lie flat on the floor, making sure you are quite warm enough and also comfortable, on a blanket or carpet. You may place a small cushion under your head if you like (not too high). Have the legs slightly apart, so that the heels are about one foot from one another and the toes relaxing gently outwards.

Now bend your arms and place the palms of your hands gently over the upper part of the rib cage, with the elbows resting lightly on the floor. As you inhale gently and to your own rhythm, feel this part of the rib cage lifting, and as you exhale, allow it to fall. Try not to involve any other part of the body in this movement. There may be a temptation to lift the shoulders or arms: resist it, not by force, but by gently letting go of any tensions here. The movement should only involve the upper rib cage.

When you have completed about half a dozen breaths to your satisfaction, change the position of the hands to the middle section of the rib cage. Now allow both upper and middle rib cage to move together, allowing more expansion of the lungs as they do so.

Next time, the hands move to the lower rib cage. Resting lightly there, feel the lung expansion filling the whole rib cage area. You may feel tempted at this stage to 'balloon' the stomach out, pushing unnaturally. Instead, simply allow the ribs to move in tune with the rhythm of the lungs. No extraneous movement need come into it! A sign that the breath is happening correctly is to position the hands so the middle fingers are just touching about 2 inches above the navel. As you breathe in, the fingers should part an inch or two by means of the rib cage movement. Exhaling brings them back together again.

It helps to have someone standing over you to see the rib cage movement, and assure you that you're increasing your lung capacity. But in the end, you're the one who has to feel it for yourself. So close your eyes, really concentrate on the sensation of a fresh stream of air entering through the nostrils, down the back of the throat and through the length of windpipe where it branches off into the bronchial tubes to be delivered and distributed throughout the lung space. Feel yourself creating space for this to happen, letting the lungs take in the air they need, and allowing the ribs encasing them to be flexible and free. As you breathe out, following the contraction of the full lung area with all the strength of the ribs, visualize all the stale air particles detaching themselves from the body, taking with them everything you no longer need — toxic waste, disease, negative thoughts. Your hands, still resting over the rib cage, gently guide its rhythmic movement.

Now that you have your own perception of the 'whole' yoga breath, with the complete rib cage allowing freedom to the lungs, it's time to go a little further. Equalize in and out breaths, each in time to a slow count of three. If you can't manage three, try a count of two; if you feel you could comfortably make it longer, do so to your own capacity. Remember, this is just as you feel most comfortable, it is not an endurance test. Gradually, though, you could extend the in and out breaths, to four or six or whatever you find best. Remember too to RELAX as you do this — just allow the breath to come and go — head, neck, shoulders, arms, tummy, legs are all left completely alone!

While you are getting used to this way of 'whole' breathing, you may like to try it on the floor for a few weeks as described; then, remember it when out walking, sitting, whenever you have the time to focus on it. It is remarkably soothing, energizing and it beats tranquillizers!

2. Only when you are completely happy with the above technique, continue to its extension. In this, the inhalation is done on a count of three; exhaling, on a count of six. You may try breathing in to four, out to eight, and so on as you feel fit! Always keep the breathing smooth. The purpose of this form of breathing is to gain greater control over breath and therefore body function. It is also relaxing. When inhaling, we draw in life and energy. Exhaling, in yoga philosophy, is an act of

humility, calming nerves and brain and bringing us into cosmic harmony. Thus, making the exhalation longer than the inhalation increases this calming, harmonizing period.

3. More advanced still, is the technique of retaining the breath between in and out breaths, or between out and in. It is, essentially, done to induce a meditational state, where the senses are stilled and the thought processes are suspended. During breath retention, say the yogic sages, we are in a state of both freedom and unity.

To try breath retention, breathe in to two, hold on a count of one, then breathe out to four (or, in to four, hold for two, out to eight). Do take care with this technique — there should be no physical or mental strain — watch heart, eyes for signs! If your rhythm of inhalation and exhalation becomes disturbed, you are over-doing things, so stop and go back to comfortable in and out breathing.

4. Alternate nostril breathing is another calming, soothing salve! Try it, sitting quietly for a few minutes, when you feel things are getting too much for you.

Sitting comfortably with the back upright and feet on the ground, lift the right hand (even if you are left-handed — the right is considered more auspicious according to ancient tradition) and tuck the fore- and middle fingers lightly into the hollow of the palm. Place the thumb to the side of the right nostril, and the ring and little fingers together beside the left nostril.

Then, pressing the thumb to close the right nostril, and lifting the ring and little fingers slightly away, breathe in for a count of four through the left nostril only. Close the left nostril with ring and little fingers then breathe out to a count of six through the right nostril.

Breathe in to a count of four through the right nostril, keeping the left one shut, then out to six through the left, shutting the right. Continue, in through one nostril then out and in through the alternate one, to the rhythm of in to four, out to six, about 15 to 20 rounds altogether (one inhalation and one exhalation makes up a round). When familiar with the exercise, you may increase the out-breath count to double that of the in-breath, as in previous breathing exercises.

This technique is useful for clearing the nasal passages (have a hanky ready!) and for making us aware of any imbalance in the use of the nostrils. An equal flow of air through both nostrils is essential for stable energy function and clarity of mind, say the ancient yogic teachings. Certainly, any nasal congestion makes for strained, irregular breathing and discomfort which may be reflected throughout the system.

5. Releasing breath. This one is great for a quick release of tension and creating general invigoration! Don't do it if you suffer from high blood-pressure, though.

Stand with legs about 2 feet apart. Clasp the hands and lift arms quickly above the head, breathing in. Then let them fall, bending forwards from the waist and swinging the hands down between the legs, relaxing the knees and also the head. As you do so, breathe out vigorously, sighing 'Ha!' as loudly as surrounding company will permit!

Chapter 6

STRETCHING SEQUENCES: THE SALUTE TO THE SUN; THE CAT

The Salute to the Sun and the Cat are two of my favourite sequences in yoga. They aren't really postures: they are a series of movements, performed in a flowing rhythm (yes, it is possible once you get the hang of it!).

I find them invaluable because even if you have no time for a full programme of yoga postures, one or both of these sequences will do nearly as much good. While they do not have the intensity of the individual postures — which are held for longer — they do give a wonderful stretch throughout the body (except for a sideways stretch).

Sun worship movements have been known throughout the centuries, and probably those incorporated into this sequence are to do with such a ritual. How they became part of the practice of yoga, no one really knows. Don't worry, though — they won't link you in mysterious ways to pagan practices! Since the sun gives life and energy to the planet, any deeper meaning in the movements is simply to do with acknowledging the power of a great and potent energy source.

This apart, however, the Salute to the Sun acts as a wonderful morning 'toner-upper' and I thoroughly recommend it to everyone. You may find the movements given here vary slightly from those seen or practised elsewhere. No matter: different teachers have their own variations and they work in virtually the same way. A few rounds of the Salute to the Sun is a great way of getting an all-round, co-ordinated, thorough stretch, and of harmonizing breathing too. Time it to suit yourself. Once you know the movements, the sequence can take a couple of minutes, or you can carry on for as long as you like! What's more you can adapt the sequence to suit how you feel. When sluggish and not at all together, do each movement slowly and painstakingly, taking care not to jerk or exert the body. If you awake full of life and vigour, a few brisk rounds will ensure that you stay invigorated.

Words don't mean much when it comes to the Salute to the Sun, though. The only way to find out just how good it is, is to go ahead and try it. And you don't even need the sun! A warm, comfortable room is the only requirement — if you're facing the rising sun, so much the better, but dark rainy mornings or long after sunrise will still have a good effect!

The pictures show two sequences. The white background is for beginners. I suggest that you study each of the twelve pictures and try out the positions one by one before moving from one to another in sequence. The pictures are only a guide. You may be able to go a little further with some of the positions (in which case, look at the dark background ones to see what to aim for). In some, you may have to do your own variation of what's shown. The point is (as with all yoga postures) to bear in mind what you're trying for, *and* to recognize what stage your body is at! You *will* gradually loosen up, and in a surprisingly short time, if you keep at it. The Salute to the Sun is a great loosener-up and even if you feel hopelessly stiff at first, with nothing but creaks and protests from your joints, do carry on as far as good sense allows (of course, any abnormal pain or stiffness will tell you when *not* to persevere, so use body awareness all the time). Although they look complex, the positions are possible, in some form, for most people, and evolving your own individual Salute to the Sun will be as valuable as doing it all 'perfectly'.

It does help to breathe in time with the movements, but this is something that comes later, when you are completely familiar with them. So don't worry about the breathing at first, just get the hang of when and where your limbs are supposed to be, and breathe naturally. When you can go into the positions without thinking too hard, gradually incorporate the breathing as you do them.

If you are using the Salute to the Sun as part of your complete yoga practice, it follows in Chapter order, that is, after your warming and limbering stretches, and the yoga breathing. By this time the body is ready for the extra stretch and is also attuned to the breathing practices, so this puts them together very nicely. If you just want to do the Salute to the Sun by itself, I recommend a warming-up stretch or two beforehand, (especially if you've just rolled out of bed,) from the limbering section, Chapter 4.

THE SALUTE TO THE SUN

Beginners

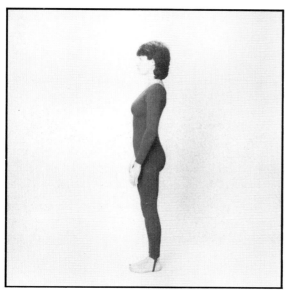

1 Stand with feet evenly on the floor, hands loosely in front of you. Close your eyes for a second and sense the equilibrium of the position. Try not to hollow the back or tense the shoulders.

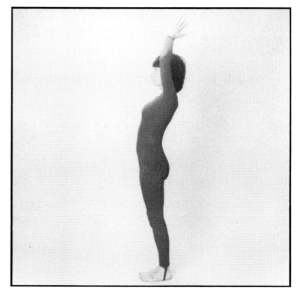

2 Breathing in, raise the arms as far as they will comfortably go, up over the head. Keep the feet firmly planted on the ground and the whole body as even as possible, without toppling to one side!

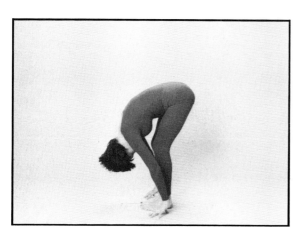

3 Breathing out, sweep the hands down, bending at the waist and knees. Allow the hands to touch the floor beside the feet if possible, and relax in this position.

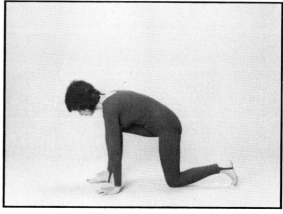

4 Breathing in, place the palms of the hands firmly on the floor in the same position as they were, beside the feet. Step back with the left foot so you are resting on the left knee, bending the right knee so you are in a crouch position.

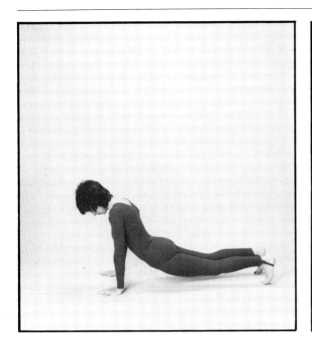

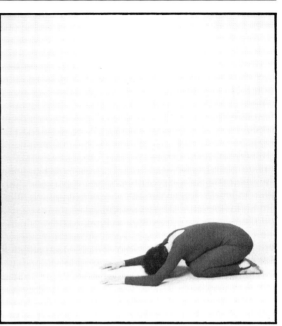

5 Breathing out, bring the left leg back behind you, resting the knee on the ground, then take the right leg back in the same position, giving a good stretch to back and legs, and resting on knees and hands.

6 Breathe in, then out, as you bend the knees further and sink back with bottom towards the heels, head towards the floor — and relax there!

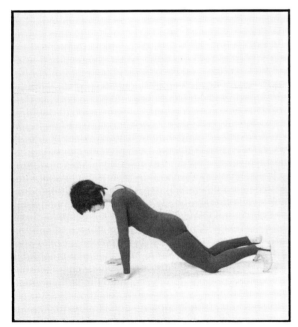

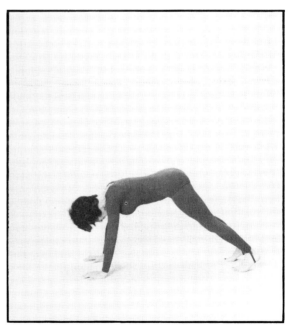

7 Breathing in, tuck toes in and raise the trunk from the ground, with knees bent and head relaxed.

8 Breathing out, push the bottom up in the air and attempt to straighten legs.

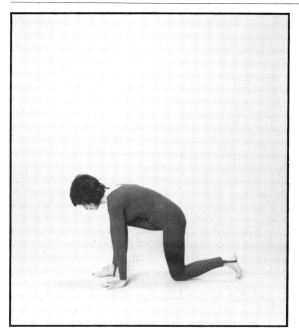

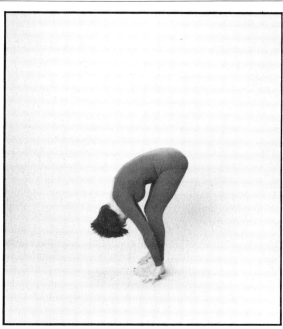

9 Breathing in, bend the left knee to the floor and step the right foot forwards between the hands.

10 Breathing out, step the left foot up beside the right and stand in the waist-bend position.

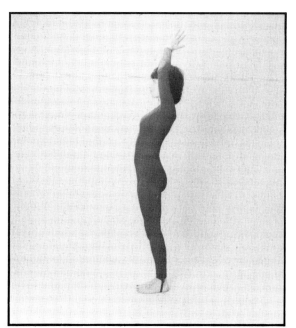

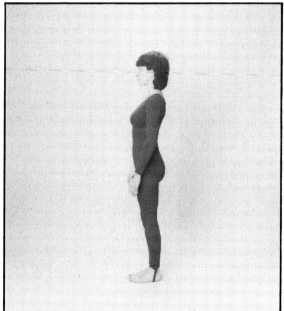

11 Breathing in, stretch up with arms over the head.

12 Breathing out, return to the straight standing position.

Recover breath and equilibrium for a few moments (you can lie on the floor and relax if you like) and then . . . begin all over again! One

'round' of the Salute to the Sun constitutes two sequences, as you have to stretch both sides equally. So this time, in step 4, bend the left knee up, with the right knee on the floor, and so on throughout the positions. Then continue, starting again with the other side, as long as you feel fit and able!

Advanced The advanced version of the Salute to the Sun, for more supple people, goes like this:

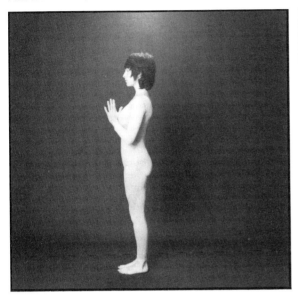

1 Stand straight, feeling firmly balanced on the floor, with palms together in front of the chest.

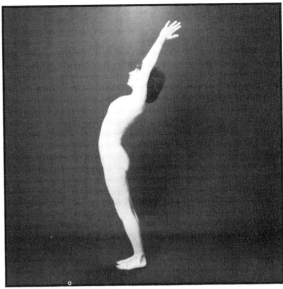

2 Breathing in, take the arms up over the head and bend back, giving a full stretch to the whole spine.

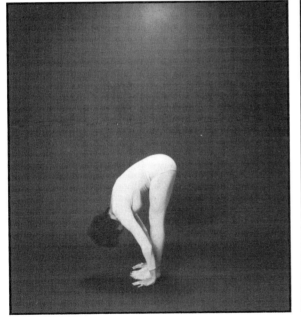

3 Breathing out, sweep the arms down, allowing the back to stretch out straight at right angles to the waist as you come down. Place hands with palms flat on the floor beside the feet and stretch the spine out as fully as possible, with legs straight.

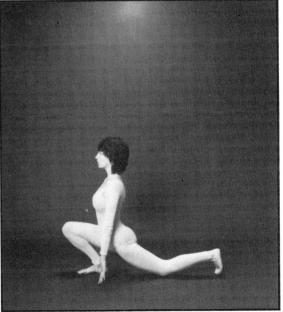

4 Breathing in, step back with the left foot, bending the right. Keep the spine as erect as possible.

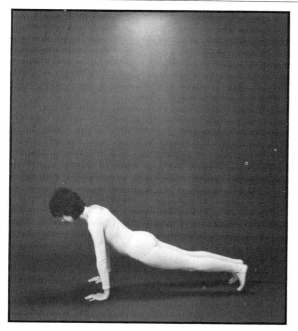

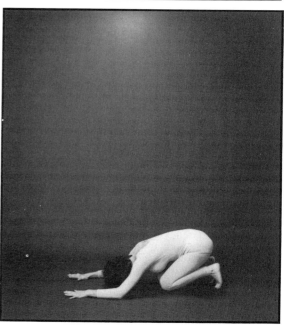

5 Breathing out, raise the left knee from the floor and place the palms on the floor, then step back with the right leg to make a straight 'plank' shape, supported by the arms.

6 Breathing in then out, place knees to the floor and sweep back so the bottom is resting on the heels.

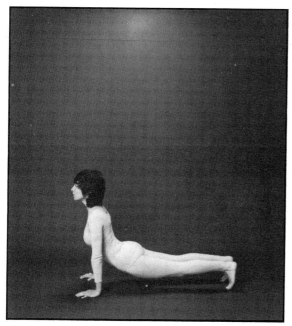

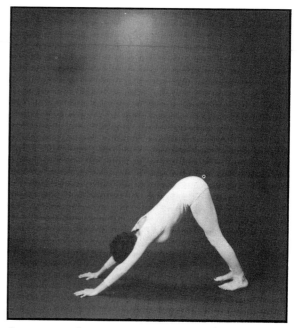

7 Breathing in, sweep the head forward, with the face as close to the ground as possible, till arms and legs are stretched and the head raised. Keep shoulders relaxed.

8 Breathing out, push the bottom back and in the air, and heels to the ground, in an inverted V-shape. Try to relax shoulders and stretch the whole spine.

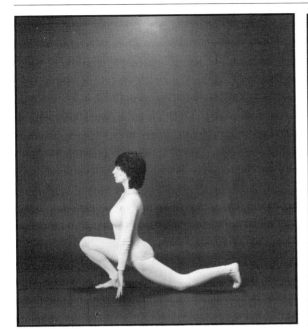

9 Breathing in, step the right foot forwards between the hands in one movement, bending the left knee, with the spine upright.

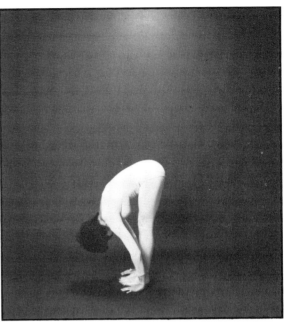

10 Breathing out, straighten the right leg and bring the left foot in, bending from the waist with palms on the floor.

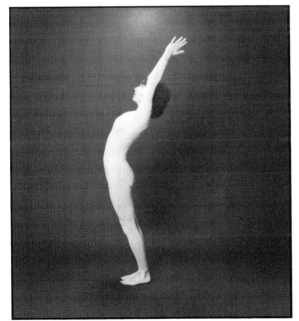

11 Breathing in, stretch up above the head.

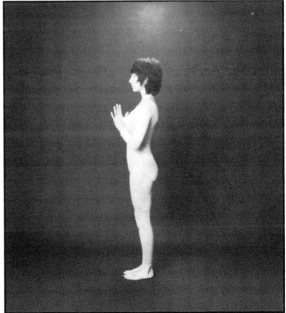

12 Breathe out as you come back to the starting position, take a few breaths with eyes closed, and repeat to the other side. Continue as long as you need!

THE CAT

The cat is a simple movement series which does just what it says — copies the fine stretching movements of the cat, to awaken and energize the spine. Do it before or after the Salute to the Sun, or on its own, any time you want to be as relaxed as a cat.

Beginners

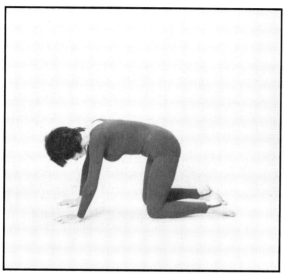

1 Kneel with legs slightly apart, hands on the floor under the shoulders. Try not to tense shoulders.

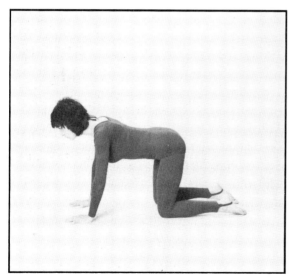

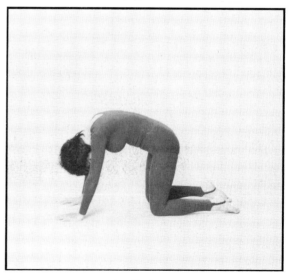

2 Raising the head and breathing in, try to 'hollow' the spine as far as possible.
3 Breathing out, lower the head as if to tuck the chin into the collar bone, and 'round' the spine as much as you can. In both movements, try to make the movement stretch all along the whole spine, not just one part of it, even though you will naturally be more flexible in one area than another. Return to starting position and relax. Repeat if you need to.

Advanced

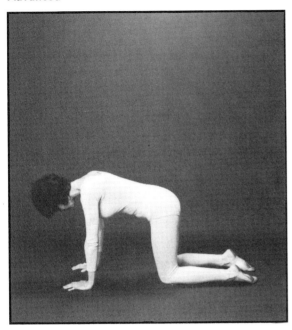

1　Kneel with legs slightly apart, hands on the floor directly under the shoulders.

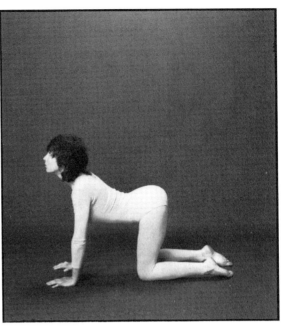

2　Raise the head as you breathe in, creating a hollow all along the spine.

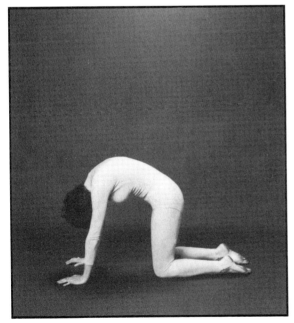

3　Breathing out, lower the head and 'round' the spine, drawing the rib cage up.

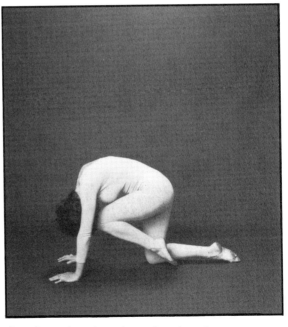

4　Take a short breath in, then breathe out as you raise the left knee to touch the forehead.

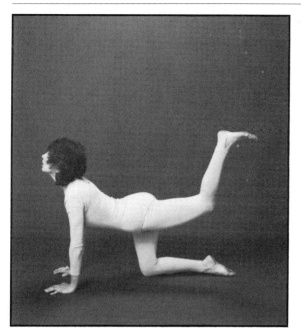 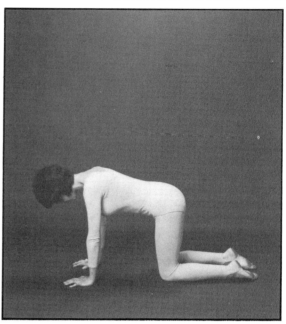

5 Breathing, stretch the left leg out behind, raising the head and hollowing out the spine, without causing undue tension on shoulders or neck.

6 Breathe out as you bring the left knee down and return to the 'all fours' starting position. Rest here and take a few breaths before repeating the sequence with the other leg.

Chapter 7

YOGA POSTURES

Now you are ready for the traditional yoga postures. It's most important to remember that the final position shown is *not* necessarily what you should be doing: it is only a guide, for you to aim towards. Start with the first black and white picture, concentrate and feel your way into the movements. If you are a beginner, instruction one may be your final posture. *It doesn't matter!* Move on when you feel strong and confident, but at all times, you are the judge of what your body needs, gaining command and taking responsibility.

The instructions are precise; again, they are to guide you into what is possible, the most constructive way of performing the postures. Suggest to your body that it attempts this way, feel and watch what happens when you try, and most important of all, don't beat yourself up, or give up, if it just doesn't want to!

Because yoga links body and mind, try out a partnership of both as you practise. It's easy to involve only one. Your mind, for example, might be telling you this is all far too complicated, or that you'll look ridiculous. Your body, on the other hand, may stretch and stiffen, or become plain lazy! So ease your mind into the postures too, gently concentrate on how they feel, what's happening as you move, allow the thoughts to rest within different areas of the body, imagine the blood flowing, the muscles releasing, the tense areas unblocking, relaxation spreading. Focus internally, on bones, connective tissues, cells — you don't have to be a biology teacher to work out what's happening where, all you need is imagination to tune into what your body is telling you!

Concentrating in this way, however you do the postures, you will be truly 'doing' yoga. What you will experience is that union between mind and body that's really at the heart of yoga practice. So again — don't worry about how far you 'get'. Just start to move, and allow yourself to focus and concentrate as you do so. There you are — doing yoga. Anyone can!

The original Sanskrit names for these postures follow the English.

1 *TREE* Vrksasana

What it does:
Increases flexibility in ankles, knees and hips.
Improves concentration.

Points to remember:
Keep your eyes on one unmoving spot in front of you to help balance.
Hip bones and shoulders should be kept level.
Bare legs help keep foot in place — it may slip against tights.
Pelvic bones should feel open.
Keep bent knee down.
Standing leg is strong.
Buttocks are held in.
Pressure from thigh keeps foot in place — keep inner thigh muscle strong!

1 Stand with one leg raised, foot against the opposite calf and hands on hips. Practise concentrating on an unmoving spot and holding the balance on one leg for a few seconds. Beginners may rest against a wall at first.

2 Place the foot higher on the opposite leg (beginners lift it with the hands) with the heel against the groin or wherever you can manage. Beginners may hold the leg in place by the ankle and attempt to find balance in this position.

3 Hands come up in the praying position, foot may be as in position 2 or across the opposite upper thigh.

Final position: Hands are in the air, palms pressed together. Draw the knee of the standing leg up 'locked' for added strength. Maintain balance for 10 seconds.

Come out: By bringing the hands down, still balancing, and then bringing the leg down. Balanced standing position before doing the other side.

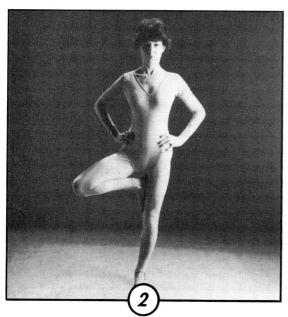

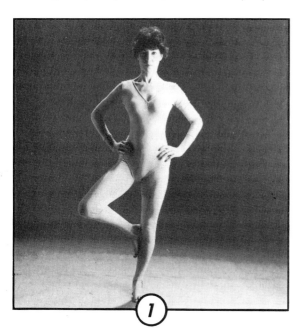

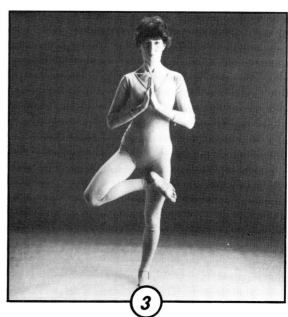

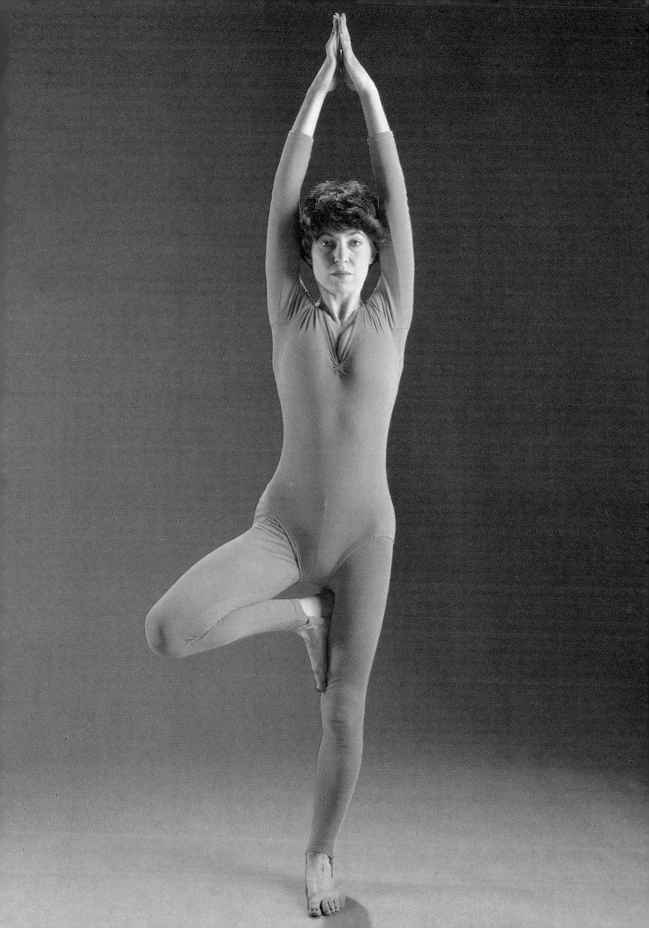

2 *WIDE LEG STRETCH* *Prasarita Padottanasana*

What it does:
Gives an intense stretch to the legs.
Stretches hips.

Points to remember:
Try initially to get your legs as wide apart as
  possible — the wider they are, the easier it is to
  balance.
Make sure you are on a non-slip surface.
Back should be straight.
The idea is not to get the head down at all costs
  — rather to stretch legs and spine. Keep weight
  on heels when bending forward — do not let
  the weight of the head pull you down.
Keep buttocks relaxed.
Keep backs of the legs taut.

1 Legs wide apart, feet facing forwards, hands on
hips.

2 Bend slightly back.

3 Now start bending forwards, hands on the tops
of the thighs.

4 Slide hands further down the legs, and stretch
out the spine, keeping the head up but not tensing
the neck.

Final position: Hands are on the floor, spine
stretched out, crown of the head on the floor
between the outstretched feet and in line with
them. Keep the position for 10 seconds.

Come out: By relaxing the back and arms, lifting
from the waist with rounded back and relaxed
head, gradually moving the feet in together and
straightening up.

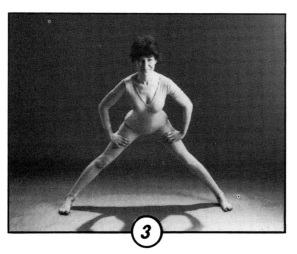

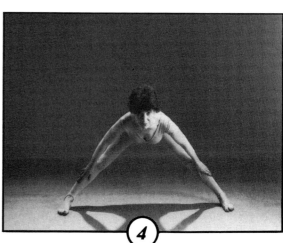

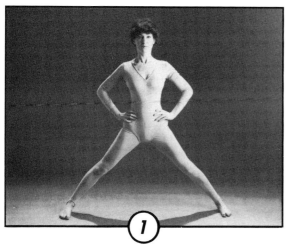

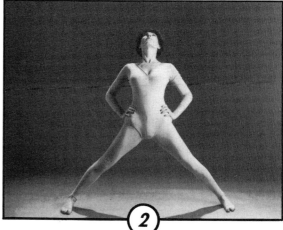

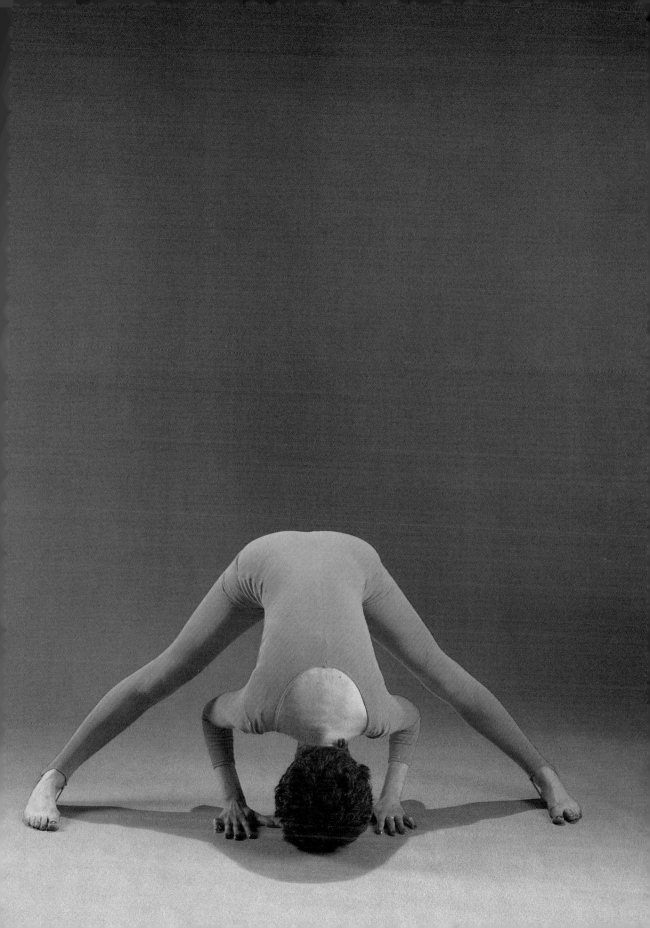

3 STANDING HEAD TO KNEE POSE
Padahastasana

What it does:
Stretches the legs and hamstrings.
Tones abdominal organs.
Helps digestion.
Helps liver and spleen activity.

Points to remember:
Keep weight evenly balanced on both feet.
Relax the buttocks and relax the whole body forwards.
Do not curve the back to move the head down —

rather, gently stretch out the whole spine for greater flexibility.

1 Keep the legs taut, and bend the torso forwards, trying to reach the floor with the fingers. If you can't reach the floor, hold as far down the legs as you can. If possible, hook the fingers underneath the toes to draw the spine out more — without tensing the shoulders or pulling! Feel the spine stretching out gently and easily.

2 Stretching the spine a little more, use the weight of the upper part of the body to stretch further forwards, trying to press the palms of the hands flat on the floor beside the feet. Legs and spine will gradually feel more flexible!

3 Holding on to the ankles, straighten the arms and look forwards, concaving the spine.

Final position: Bring the elbows behind the knees, still holding behind ankles, and push out the backs of the knees to ensure legs are kept straight. Attempt to lay chest and stomach on to the thighs and head to knees without tensing the back of the neck or shoulders. Stay 10 seconds.

Come out: By relaxing the back and head, bringing the arms loosely to sides, and straightening up from the waist, 'uncurling' vertebra by vertebra from waist to neck, finally bringing the head upright.

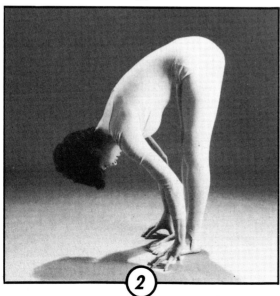

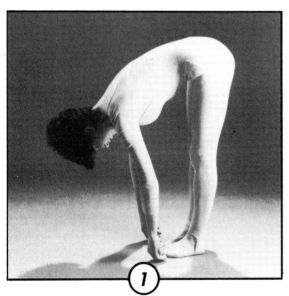

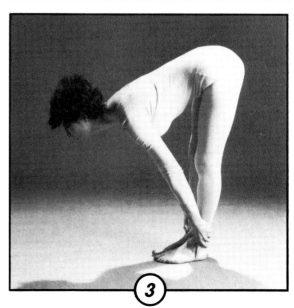

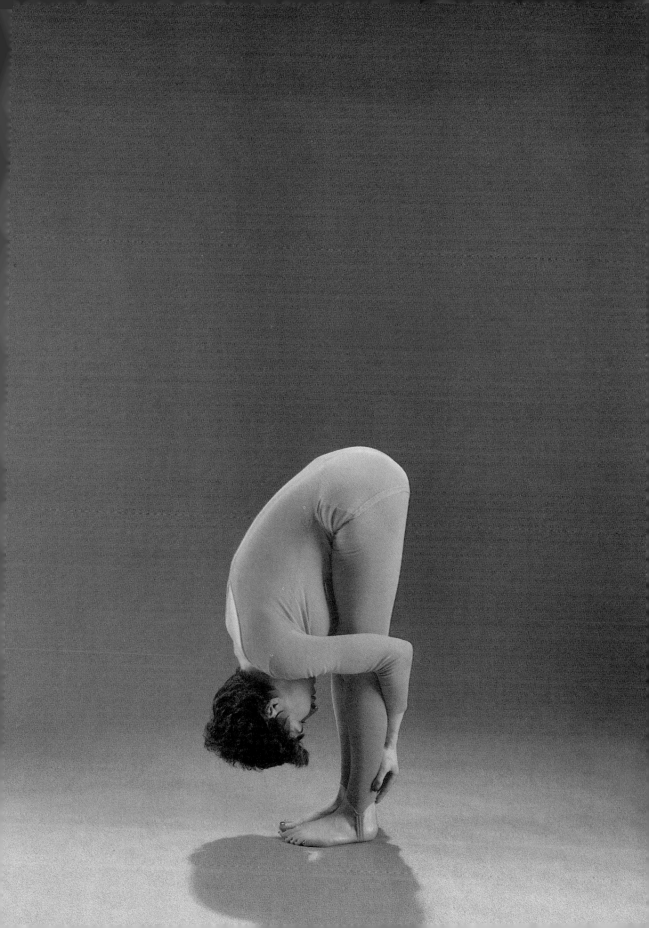

4 *WARRIOR POSE 1* *Virabhadrasana 1*

Not recommended for people with heart conditions.

What it does:
Expands the chest.
Helps deep breathing.
Relieves stiff shoulders.
Tones ankles and knees.

Points to remember:
Keep outstretched (back) leg straight.
Upper part of the body should be facing directly forwards.
Keep hips in line with each other.
Thigh of the bent (front) leg should form a right angle with the floor.
This is a strong posture, so don't be disheartened if you find it strenuous!

1 Stand with feet 4 ft apart (or as far as you can manage; turn the right foot in, left foot out, pivot round and place hands on waist. 'Lock' the knees and concentrate on keeping the legs firm. Relax the shoulders.

2 Bend the front leg, attempting a right angle. Keep the back leg straight and firm!

3 Stretch the arms up above the head, palms pressed together, as straight as they will go.

Final position: Look up at the outstretched hands, stretching the spine. Stay in position for 10 seconds.

Come out: Straighten the back and leg, bring hands down to sides, face the front keeping feet apart, pivot round to the other side and repeat.

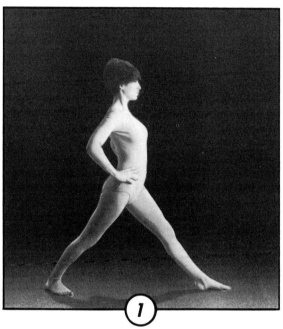

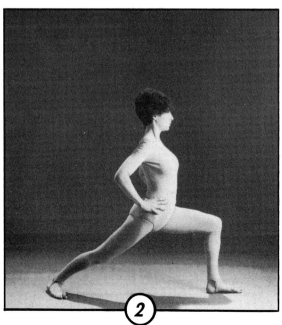

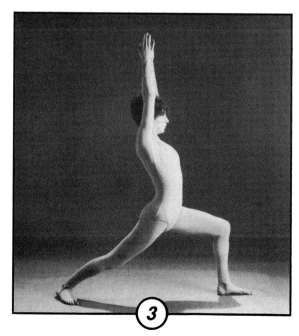

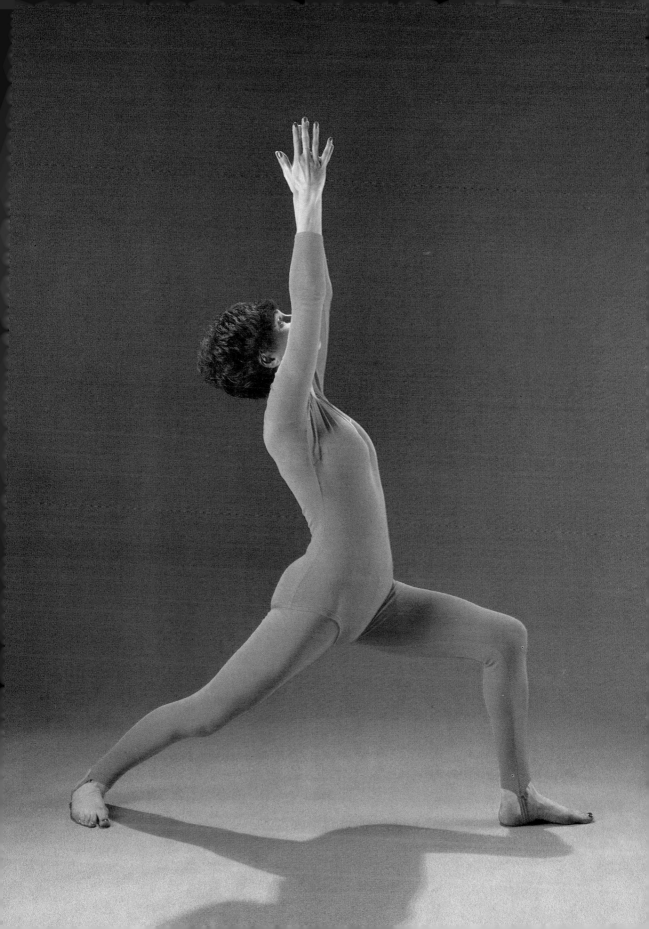

5 WARRIOR POSE 2 *Virabhadrasana 2*

Do not attempt this posture if you have a heart condition.

What it does:
Strengthens the leg muscles.
Improves suppleness of legs.
Tones abdominal organs.
Strengthens will-power and determination.

Points to remember:
Outstretched leg should be kept straight.
Bent leg should attempt a right angle.
Keep shoulders and neck relaxed.
Feel as if the hands are being pulled in opposite directions.
Expand chest.
Sink down as if sitting into the posture.
Keep torso as upright as possible.

1 Stand with feet 4 ft apart (less for beginners), right foot out, left foot slightly in. Stretch arms and fingers.

2 Turn your head to the right, keeping the chest facing forwards.

3 Begin to bend the right leg, feeling strong and balanced in the position.

Final position: Leg bent, arms outstretched, look to the right hand, keeping the legs fully stretched and the hips in line with each other. Stay 10 seconds.

Come out: Straighten leg, turn to face forwards, turn feet to face the opposite direction and repeat the posture.

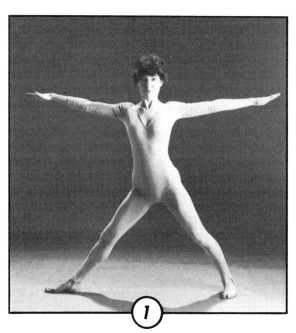

1

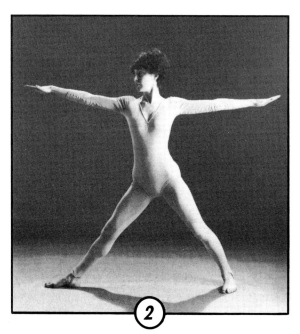

2

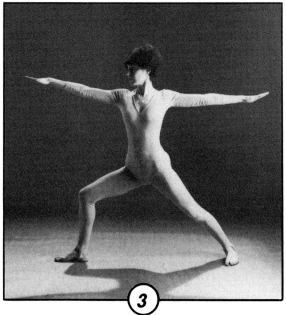

3

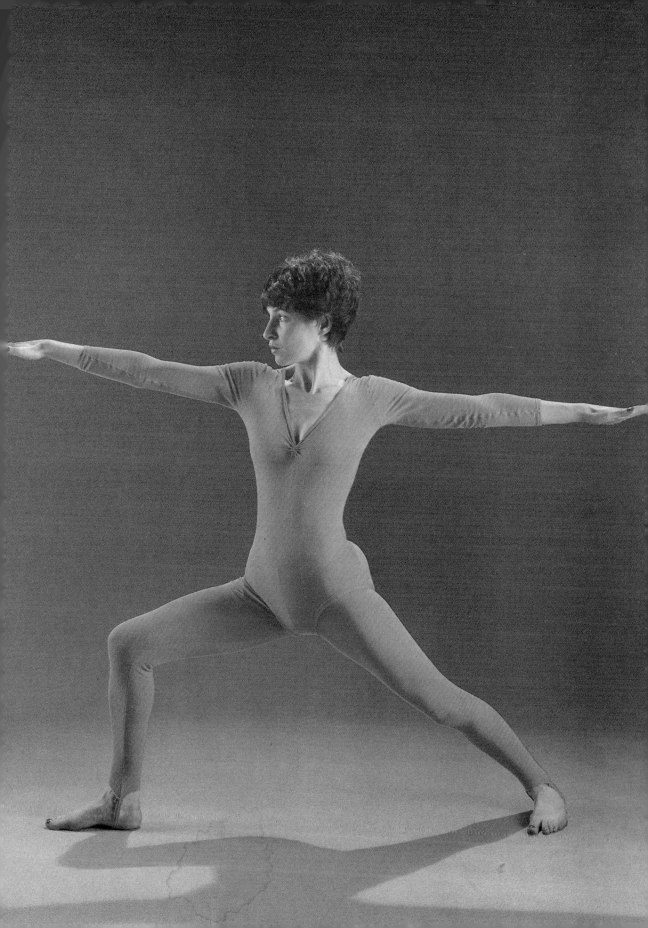

6 *SIDEWAYS LEG STRETCH* Parsvottanasana

What it does:
Helps to make legs and hips more supple.
Contracts and thus tones abdominal organs.
Relieves tense shoulders.

Points to remember:
Keep knees 'locked' to straighten legs.
Upper part of body should face directly forward.
Hips should be in line with each other.

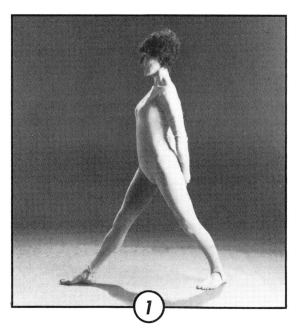

Keep upper part of the body in line while going down — do not twist to side.
Balance weight equally on both feet — and on both sides of the ankles.
Keep torso lengthened and extend along thigh while going down.
Aim is not to get head to knee, but to lengthen upper body along thigh.

1 Stand with feet about 3 ft apart. Turn right foot out, left foot slightly in. Hands are lightly clasped just below the buttocks. Body is facing sideways, chest expanded, shoulders back and down, buttocks tucked in. Feel the strength in the legs.

2 Bend back slightly, drawing the hands down. Feel the spine becoming more flexible, the legs straight.

3 Begin to come forward with straight back, weight balanced in the legs.

Final position: Bring the hands up over the head, weight still on both feet, as if the chest is going to meet the thigh. Head is relaxed. Stay for 10 seconds.

Come out· By lowering the hands to the lower back, swinging the trunk round hips, turning feet in the opposite direction, and thus bending over the other leg. Stay 10 seconds, lower hands, raise torso, face forwards, bring feet together.

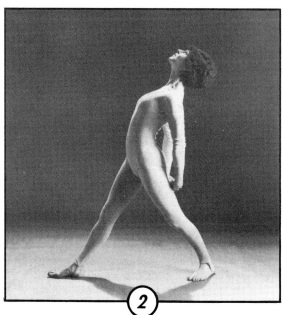

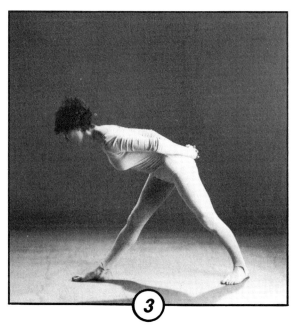

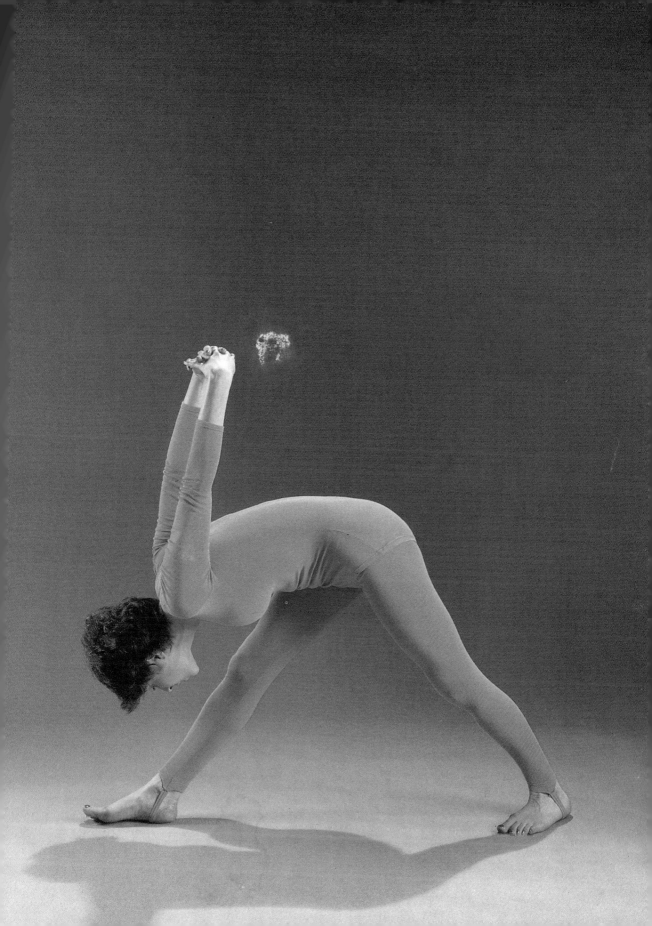

7 *TRIANGLE* *Trikonasana*

What it does:

An 'all purpose' stretch, toning the whole body.
Particularly good for toning leg muscles, and improving strength and flexibility of the hip joint.
Stretches sides of the torso.
Firms chest muscles.

Points to remember:

Keep standing legs absolutely straight.
Thighs should push away from each other.
Hips should widen away from one another.
Outstretched side should feel soft — not tense — while stretching.
Chest should feel 'open' and on one plane — as if the torso were sandwiched between two boards.

1 Feet about 3 ft apart, right foot turned out, left foot slightly inwards. Hands on hips. Top half of the body should face forwards.

2 Slide the right hand down the leg, bending the sides of the body, feeling the stretch in the left side.

3 Hand slides down towards the ankle, upper shoulder is drawn back, head looking up.

Final position: Left arm raised, looking up to the outstretched hand. Remain for 15 seconds.

Come out: By looking down at the ankle, lifting the downstretched arm, bringing both arms out to the sides as you raise the torso, dropping the arms and bringing the feet to face forwards. Repeat on the other side.

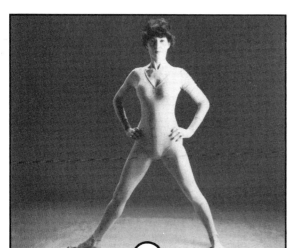

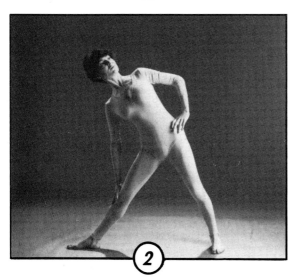

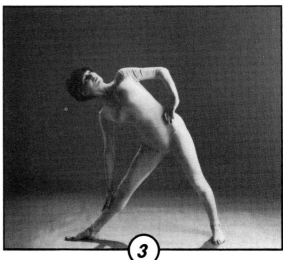

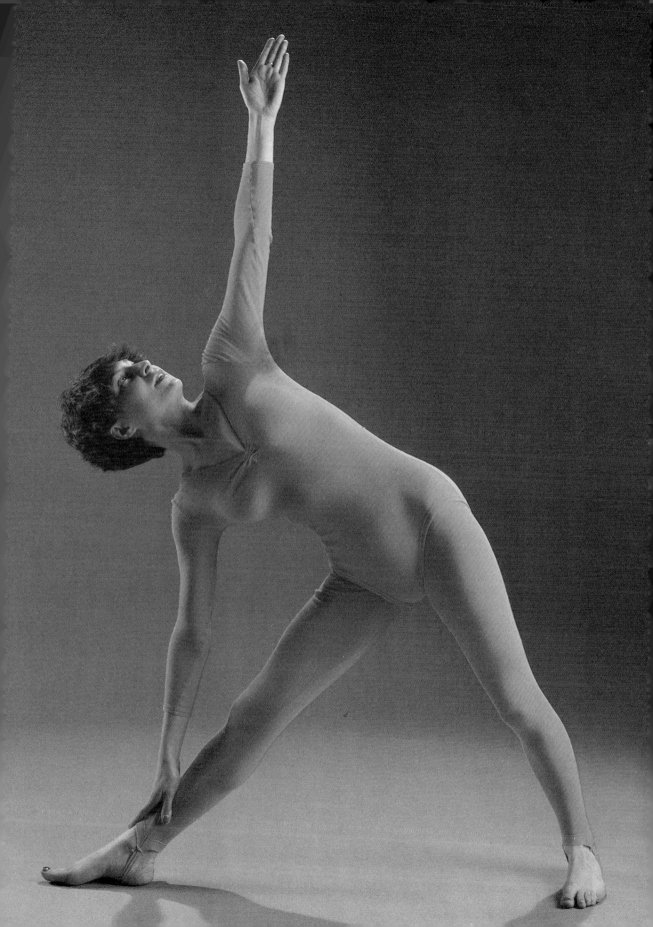

8 *GATE* *Parighasana*

What it does:
Tones and flexes the sides of the torso.

Points to remember:
Keep the neck soft.
No tension in the shoulders.
Stretch out from the thigh to the fingertips.
Trunk remains in one place; do not tilt.
Outstretched leg stays straight and firm.

1 Kneel on right leg; stretch out the left leg to the side, foot facing forward, toes in line with the opposite knee. Hands on hips. Feel yourself stretching from the legs upwards; keep the shoulders down.

2 Right arm stretches up, left hand rests on thigh. Again, the feeling is of a complete stretch all the way along the right side of the body — easing out rather than pulling.

Final position: Allow the outstretched arm to rest close to the right ear and the whole of the right side to stretch. Stay for 10 seconds.

Come out: By bringing the arm up again and straightening the torso, bringing the arms to the sides and kneeling on both knees. Repeat on the other side.

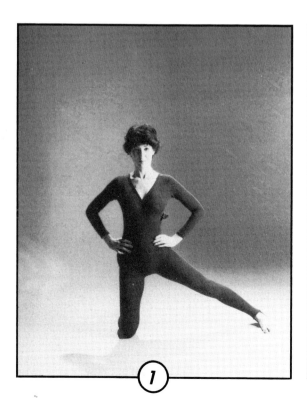

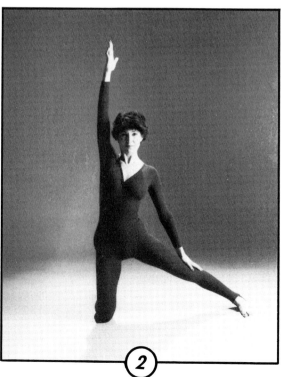

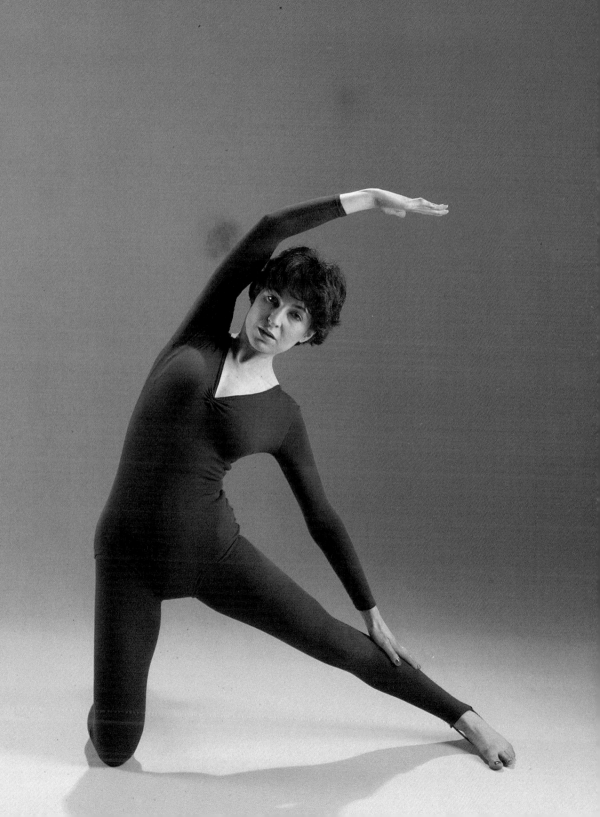

9 **CAMEL** *Ustrasana*

What it does:
Stretches the abdominal organs.
Stretches front thighs.
Tones throat, thyroid and parathyroid glands.
Opens rib cage.
Improves flexibility of spine and neck.
Tones muscles of abdomen.

Points to remember:
Concentrate on the knees to waistline.
Thrust pelvis forward in order to arch back.
Relax the small of the back.

1   Start the posture by kneeling — beginners may have the knees apart.

2   Stretch out the thighs, holding them for support, and bend the back as far as is comfortable. Get the feeling of elongating the thighs and contracting the back. Relax head by lengthening from base of neck and allowing it to go back as far as is comfortable.

Final position: Hands on heels, hips pushed forwards, with a strong stretch to the thighs. Back is arched, head relaxed. Stay for 10 seconds.

Come out: By bending the arms and sinking back on to the heels — then bring the head to the floor, arms to either side, stretching the small of the back and easing out the previous contraction.

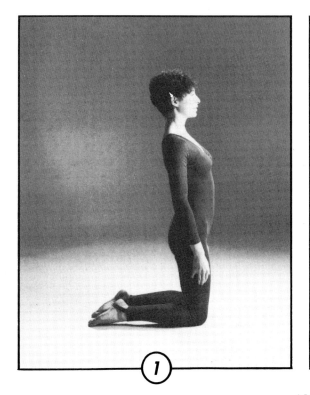
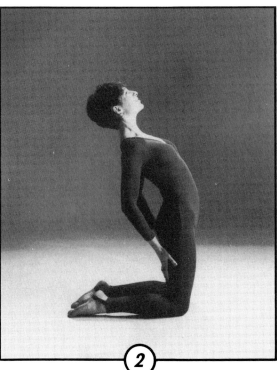

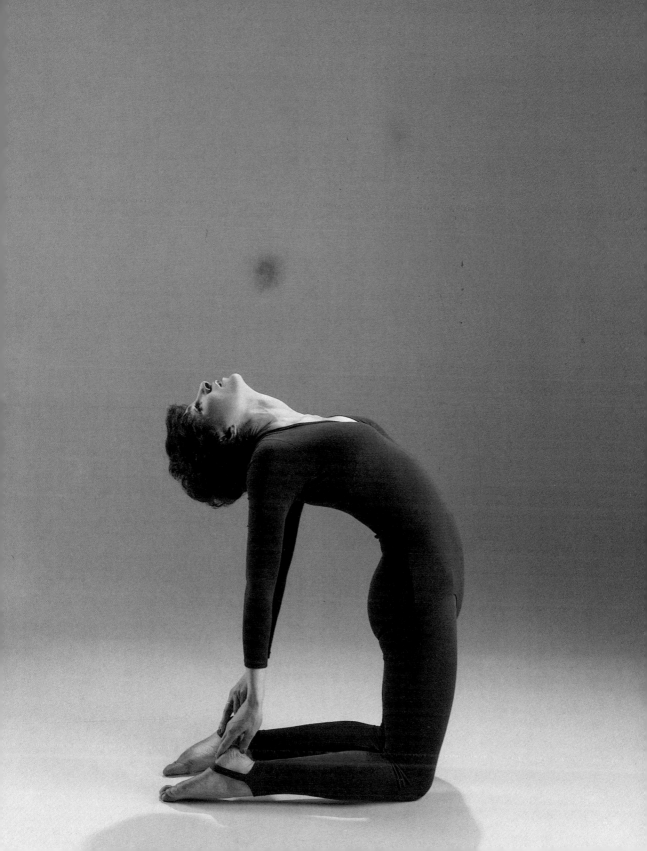

10 *FORWARD BEND* Paschimottanasana

What it does:
Tones the whole spinal column.
Strengthens abdominal organs.
Massages the heart.
Helps action of the kidneys.
Improves digestion.
Tones sexual organs.

Points to remember:
The object is to stretch out the spine — not to bend forwards to get the head on the knees.
The movement should take place from the pelvis and waist.
Do not pull from the shoulders; arms should stay relaxed and only be used as supports.
'Props' can be used to guide the spine downwards.
Legs should stay straight — push backs of knees down to prevent bending!

1 Sit on the floor with legs straight out in front of you, toes up. Spread the flesh of the buttocks outwards to give you a relaxed 'seat' from which to bend forwards. Begin to bend slightly from the waist, keeping the back straight.

2 Using a belt or tie round the feet, gently guide the upper part of the body down over the legs.

3 Bend further down along the legs. Stretch spine out further to get into the closing jack-knife position.

Final position: Bend as far as you can over the legs, without bending at the knees or rounding the shoulders and back. Try to relax the tummy on to the thighs and the face on the knees. Stay for 10 seconds.

Come out: By relaxing and rounding the back and sitting upright.

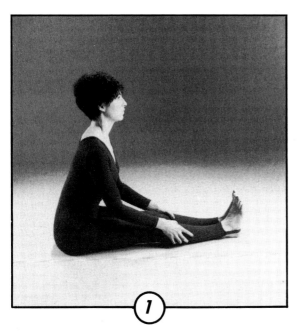

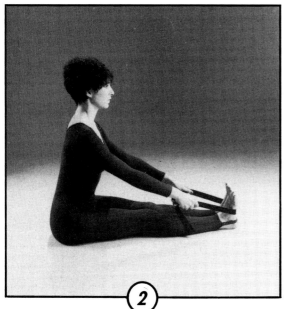

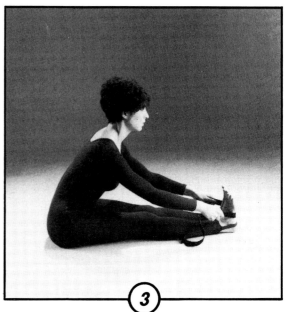

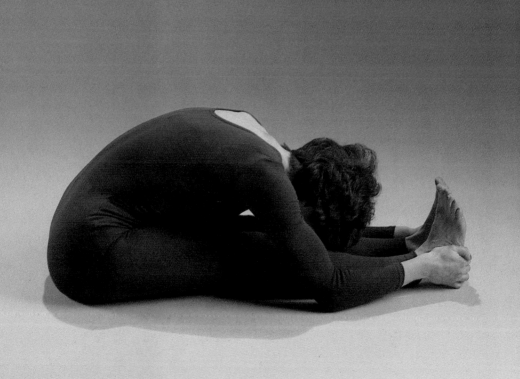

11 FORWARD BEND OVER ONE LEG
Janu Sirsasana

What it does:
Tones liver and spleen.
Aids digestion.
Activates kidneys.

Points to remember:
Extended leg should remain straight.
Spine should stretch out over the outstretched leg,
    as with the Forward Bend.
Stretch both sides of the body equally over the leg;
    do not be tempted to pull one side down at the
    expense of the other!

1 Sit on the floor with one leg outstretched, knee
pushed down. The other knee is bent out to the
side with foot pressed against the top of the
opposite thigh.

2 Still keeping the outstretched leg straight,
gently push the other knee down towards the floor,
with the spine erect.

3 Using a belt or tie, persuade the upper body
down towards the outstretched leg, keeping it
facing forwards and stretching evenly. The bent
knee should remain as near the floor as possible
with most of the initial stretch coming from the
waist and pelvis.

4 Take hold of the toes and bring the body
further forwards.

Final position: Reach down over the leg with even
stretch throughout the upper body, the toes of the
straight outstretched leg upright and the buttocks
evenly balanced and relaxed on the floor. Stay 10
seconds.

Come out: By relaxing the hold on the toes,
coming to an upright position and stretching out
the bent leg; bounce both legs up and down for a
moment, then repeat to the other side.

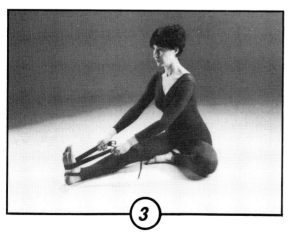
1

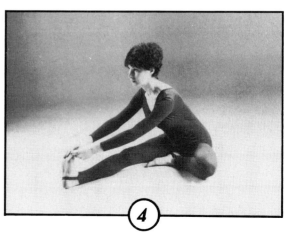
2

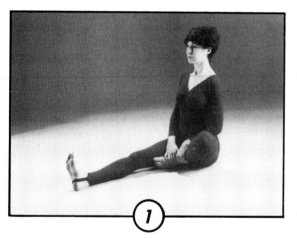
3

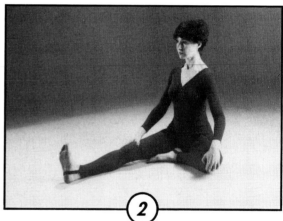
4

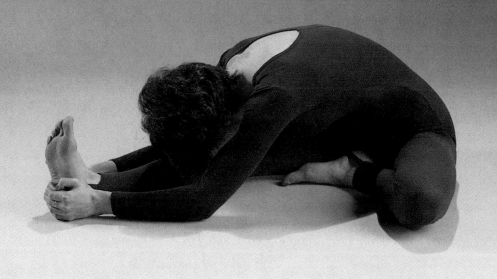

12 **COBRA** *Bhujangasana*

What it does:
Tones the whole spine.
Expands the chest.
May help menstrual problems.
Corrects bad posture.
Improves function of liver and spleen.
Strengthens deltoid and trapezius muscles.
Tones adrenal glands.

Points to remember:
The strength in this posture comes from the back
   itself — so don't rely on the arms; they are only
   'extra' supports.
Do not hunch the shoulders!
Do not tense buttocks.

1   Lie on your front on the floor, toes out, hands
palms down and fingers in line with the shoulders.
Forehead is on the floor.

2   Gently slide the chin to the spot where the
forehead was, thus beginning the curve to the
upper spine.

3   Now raise the chest off the floor, using the
arms for support as little as possible, but using the
strength and vitality of the spine.

4   Raise up higher, this time using the arms but
not relying too heavily on them. Keep the pelvic
area on the floor, and the shoulders relaxed; feel
the gentle elongation and curving of the spine.

Final position: Stretch further, look upwards (like a
cobra!), releasing the small of the back while
pushing the tummy down on to the floor. Stay for
10 seconds.

Come out: By bending the arms and letting the
upper body down gently to the floor. You may sit
back on your heels, with your head to the floor, if
you need to stretch out the lower back.

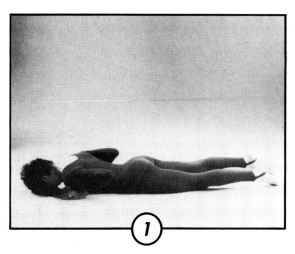

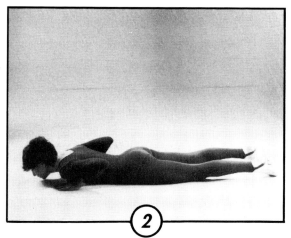

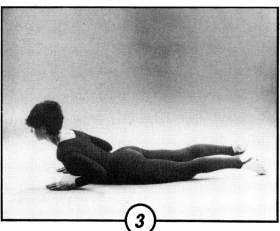

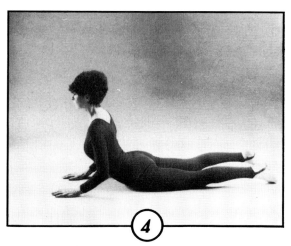

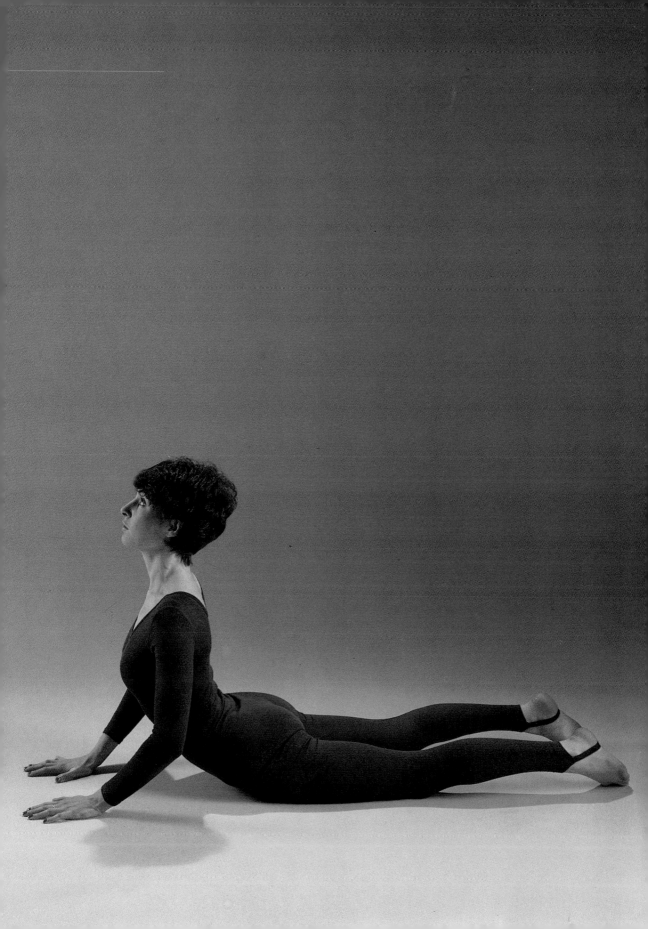

13 LOCUST *Salabhasana*

Do not do this pose if you have high blood-pressure.

What it does:
Makes spine more supple.
Helps back and spinal problems, especially in the lower back.
Benefits the bladder.
Strengthens lungs and respiratory system.
Activates the adrenal glands.
Firms buttocks and hips.

Points to remember:
Try to concentrate on the muscles of the lower back and the abdomen to lift the legs off the ground.
Pressing the floor hard with hands and arms helps to lift the legs.
Do not tilt to one side when lifting each leg separately.
Do not tense shoulder or facial muscles.

1 Lie face down on the floor and concentrate on the lower back — this is the area you will use to do the lifting.

2 Place the chin on the floor, and clench the hands underneath the thighs. Use the muscles of the lower back to lift one leg straight in the air. The hip of the raised leg should remain touching the forearm; the other hip and leg are on the ground. Keep the muscles of the locked leg taut. Stay in this position (the half-locust) for 2 seconds, then lower the leg gently to the floor and relax the arms, shoulders and legs.

3 Repeat with the other leg.

4 Hands may be clenched with palms facing up or down, whichever you find most comfortable. Same position as before, with chin on the floor. Lift both legs together, again concentrating on the lower back muscles to provide energy. Stay for 2 seconds, lower legs gently and under control to the floor.

Final position: Both legs and upper part of the body are lifted in the air, with the arms outstretched for support.

Come out: By lowering gently and in a controlled way to the floor, as before, trying to get feet and head to reach the floor at the same time. Then rest with the legs slightly apart, arms out at the sides, and the face turned on one cheek.

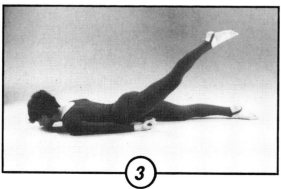

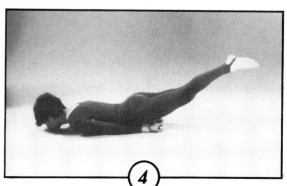

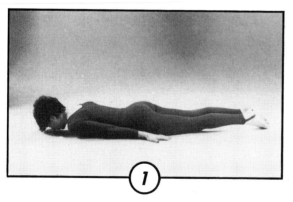

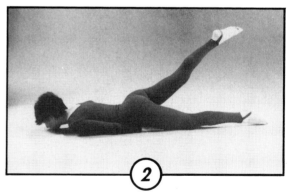

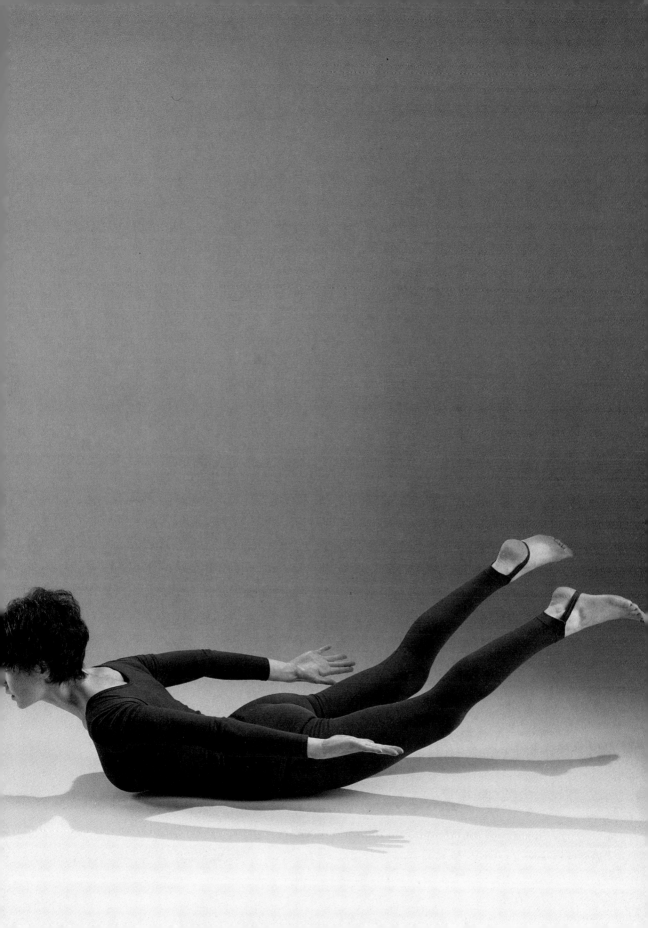

14 BOW Dhanurasana

What it does:

Helps make the spine supple.

Tones abdominal organs including liver, kidneys, spleen.

Opens rib cage.

Points to remember:

Grip the feet firmly.

Concentrate on the small of the back and the buttocks in order to obtain the lift; the abdomen should push down into the floor.

Do not tug at the legs with your arms; movement comes from the spine with arms only as secondary support and as light and relaxed as possible.

Do not pull on the shoulders.

1 Lie face down on the floor, bend knees and grip firmly round the feet. Make sure there is a good stretch on the front of the thighs.

2 With knees a hip width apart, gently raise the thighs off the ground by using the strength in the lower back.

3 Raise the head and legs off the ground.

Final position: Legs and upper torso are raised off the ground by the strength of the back, with the abdomen the centre of balance. Stay for 5 seconds.

Come out: By gently lowering legs and chest, letting go of the feet, and resting with one cheek on the floor. You may then sit back on the heels and rest the head in front on the floor, easing out the lower back.

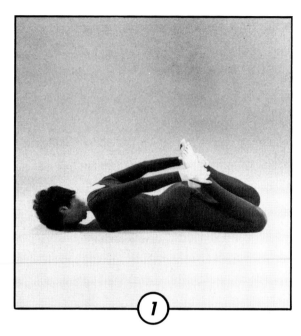

①

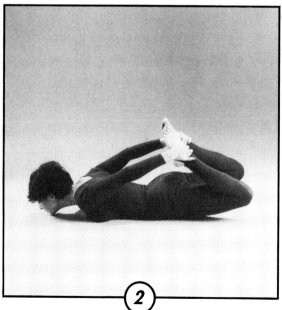

②

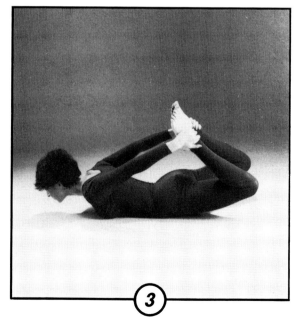

③

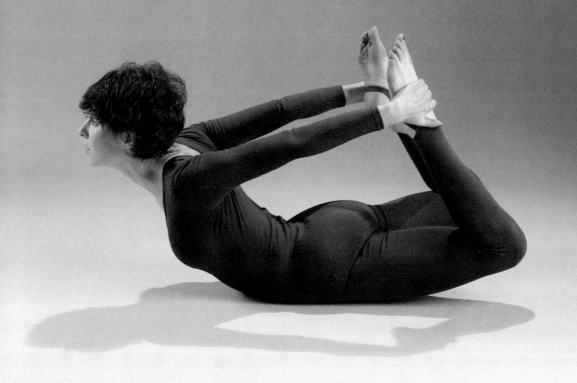

15 **DOG** *Adho Mukha Svanasana*

What it does:
Energizes the body.
Strengthens the legs.
Eases the shoulders.
Creates suppleness in the upper spine.
Strengthens the abdominal muscles.
Slows the heart rate.

Points to remember:
Work towards pressing the heels down.
Keep the back straight.
Press shoulder blades down and away from each
   other.
Do not tense buttocks.
Keep neck relaxed.
Flatten palms and fingers on the floor.

1   Kneel with thighs vertical, back straight and
palms on the floor, pressing your weight down to
straighten fingers.

2   Come up on the toes and hands, keeping legs
straight. You may practise this position with the
heels against the wall for support.

Final position: Body is in an upturned 'V' position,
heels down, front of shoulders pushing down, legs
taut.

Come out: By kneeling then sitting back on the
heels.

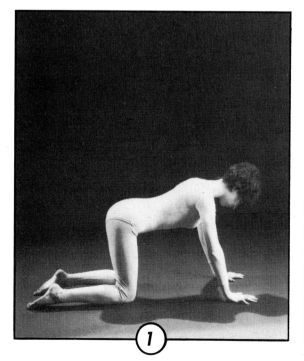

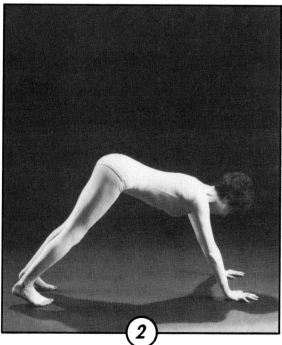

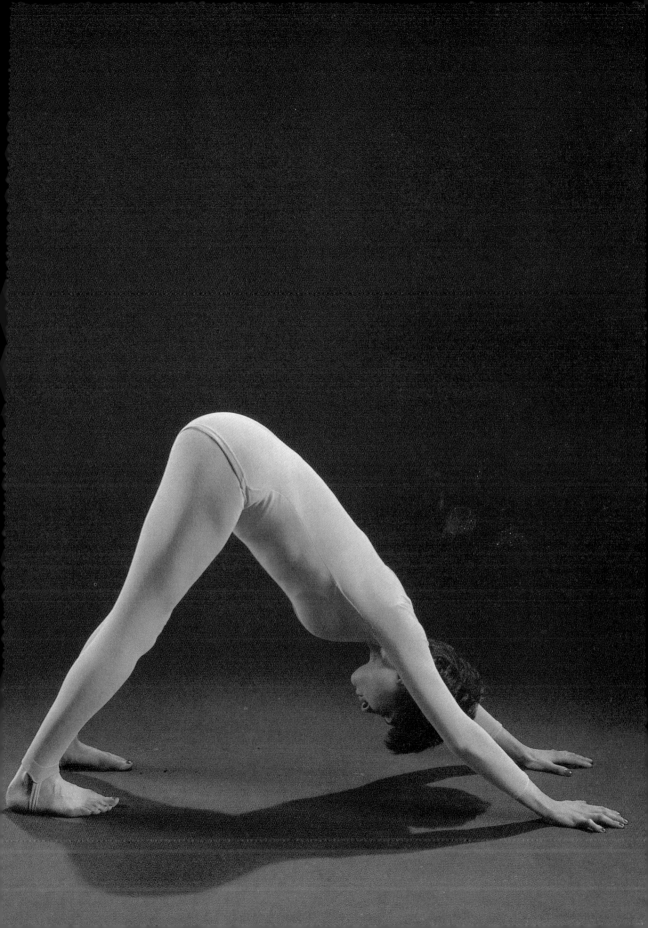

16 *LEG RAISING* *Urdhva Prasarita Padasana*

People with back problems should not attempt the full position until perfectly comfortable with the preliminary positions.

What it does:
Strengthens and tones abdominal muscles.
Strengthens lower back.
Tones leg muscles.

Points to remember:
The lower back area (behind the waist) should retain contact with the floor — make sure not to over-hollow here.
Keep shoulders on the floor.
Keep face and eyes relaxed.
Keep legs straight in the final position.
Feet are flat in final position.

1   Lie on the back, arms to the sides, palms facing down, knees bent. Relax the shoulders and press the small of the back into the floor.

2   Clasp round the knees, bringing the back further into contact with the floor.

3   Place arms back to the floor beside you. Swing the legs up, with bent knees and palms facing down.

4   Straighten the legs at a slight angle to the body, holding round the thighs for support. Feel the back pressing into the floor.

5   Straighten the legs until they reach a right-angle with the upper body, still supporting them with the hands.

6   After holding the final position, lower the legs gently to the floor, keeping them straight and keeping the back pressed against the floor.

Final position: Legs unsupported at right angles to the body, arms down, back flat against the floor. Stay for 10 seconds.

Come out: Either by bending the knees and gently straightening out on the floor, or as in 6, lowering the straight legs gradually and under control. After which, you may raise the legs, and lower them, as many times as you wish! (Maximum 10).

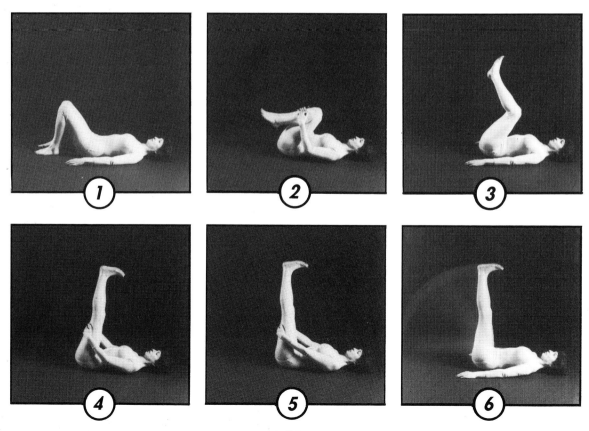

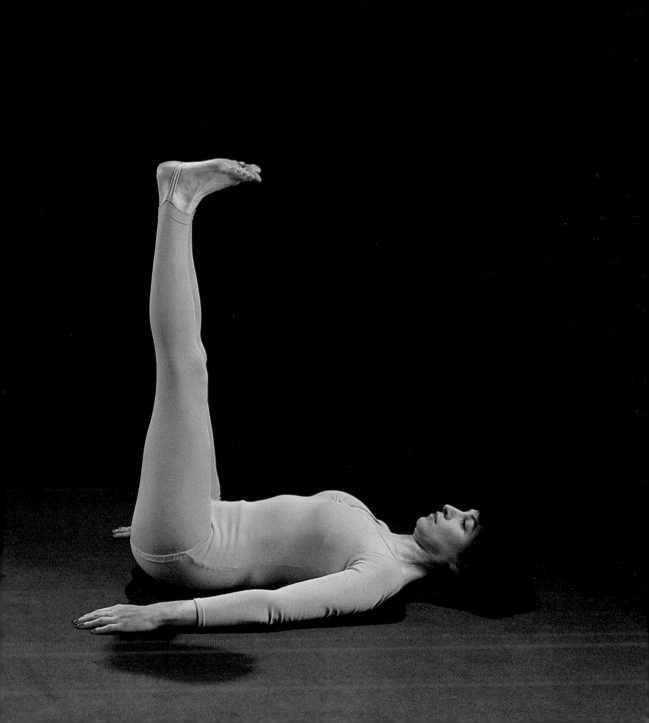

17 **HEADSTAND** *Sirsasana*

Do not do this posture if you suffer from glaucoma, detached retina, extreme short-sightedness, high blood-pressure, Ménière's disease, if you have suffered concussion or during menstruation.

What it does:
Reverses blood flow, so helps circulation.
Helps activate pineal and pituitary glands.
Relieves constipation.
Energizes and activates the whole body.
Aids balance.
Helps concentration and will-power.

Points to remember:
The headstand is not particularly difficult, but you should be reasonably fit and strong before attempting it, and also, preferably, used to some of the other postures. Practise the leg raising to help.

Abdominal tone and back strength help with headstand.

Weight should be on the top-most point of the head with neck straight.

The body should feel light in the final position.

There should be no strain in neck or shoulders — do not 'crush' the neck.

Legs should be well stretched with a sense of equal balance throughout the body.

1 Kneel with the head on a firm, but comfortable, support. The clasped hands lightly cradle the back of the head. Elbows are the same distance apart as the outstretched clasped hands. If you feel discomfort at any time, do not continue.

2 Raise your bottom in the air and stretch the legs out straight.

Keep shoulders relaxed and hands lightly clasped without clenching the fingers. Start to feel the point of balance on the head.

3 Walk the feet in towards the head, keeping arms and hands in position and straightening the back, until you feel your feet are just about to come off the ground.

4 Bend the knees and push feet off the ground by using the strength of the back and abdominal muscles.

5 Bring the thighs gradually to vertical, keeping knees bent.

Final position: Whole body vertical and evenly balanced, constantly adjusting to feel light and more upright and prevent sagging or tension especially around the neck, shoulders and upper back. Hold for as long as you are able!

Come out: By bending the knees into the chest and coming down under control until you are kneeling with face down. People who are very strong may try coming down with straight legs, bending at an angle from the waist. Remain in this position for several seconds, until breathing is normal and there is no dizziness, then come to a seated kneeling position and roll the head gently once or twice in each direction.

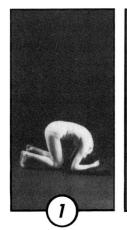
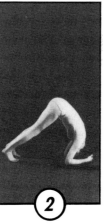
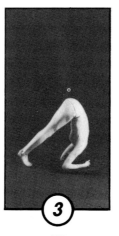
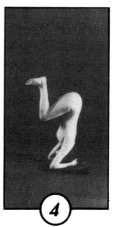
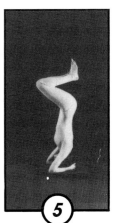

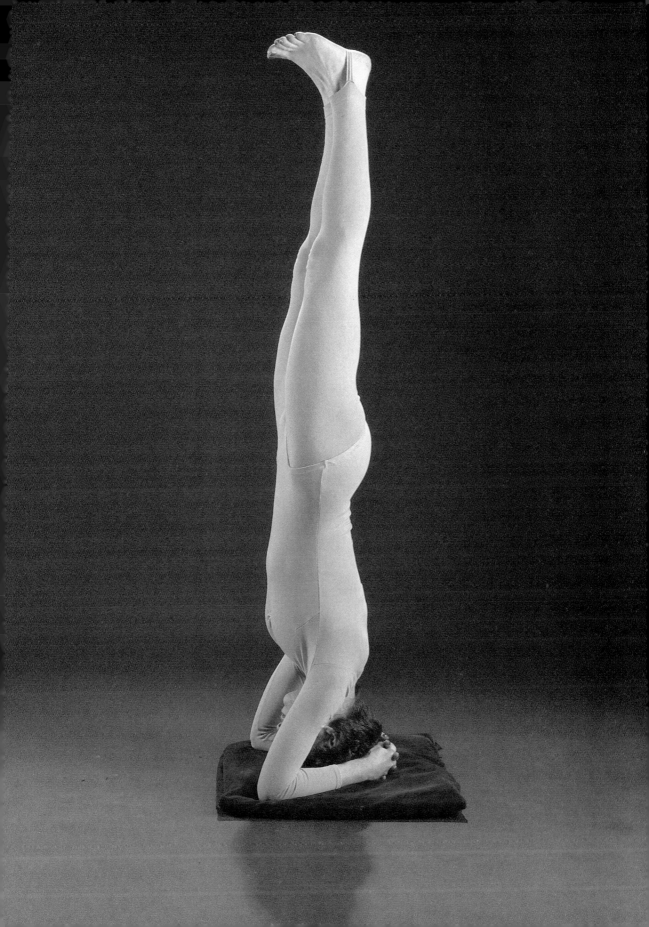

18 *SHOULDERSTAND* *Sarvangasana*

Do not do this posture during the first few days of a menstrual period.

What it does:
Tones hormones and endocrine system, particularly the thyroid and parathyroid glands.
Reverses blood flow.
Strengthens activity of the heart.
Energizes and revitalizes the whole system.
Soothes the nerves.
Increases confidence.

Points to remember:
Keep elbows well in.
Tuck chin into collar bone hollow.
Attempt to raise yourself high so the balance is taken on the shoulders rather than the upper back.
Beginners should have a chair ready for support.

1 Lie on the back with knees bent and arms out to the sides, lengthening out the back of the neck and pushing the small of the back into the floor.
2 Raise the bottom off the floor, supporting it with your hands, beginning to feel that you are shifting the balance towards the shoulders.

3 Straighten the legs out behind you, resting the feet on a chair and supporting the back with your hands. Press the torso gently into a vertical position.

4 Raise the feet higher, still supporting the back.

5 Begin to come further up on to the shoulders, with the body almost in a vertical position.

Final position: Legs are straight, the body balanced on the shoulders, hands supporting the back, chin towards the chest. Stay for 20 seconds.

Come out: By bringing the knees to the forehead, lowering the arms to the floor, and uncurling the spine along the floor vertebra by vertebra until you're lying flat again. If the back of the neck feels stiff, massage it gently, then tilt the head back with shoulders and upper back off the floor, and crown of the head on the floor for a few seconds.

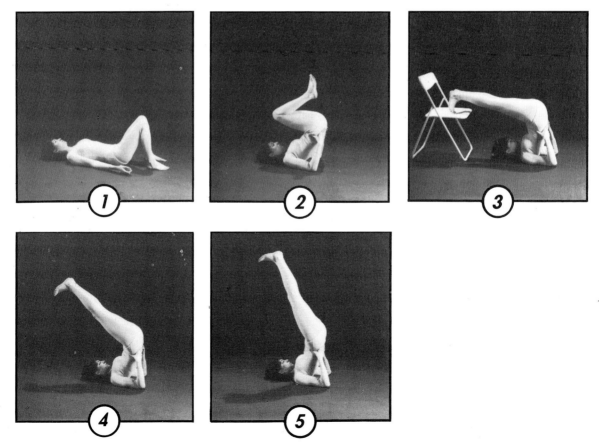

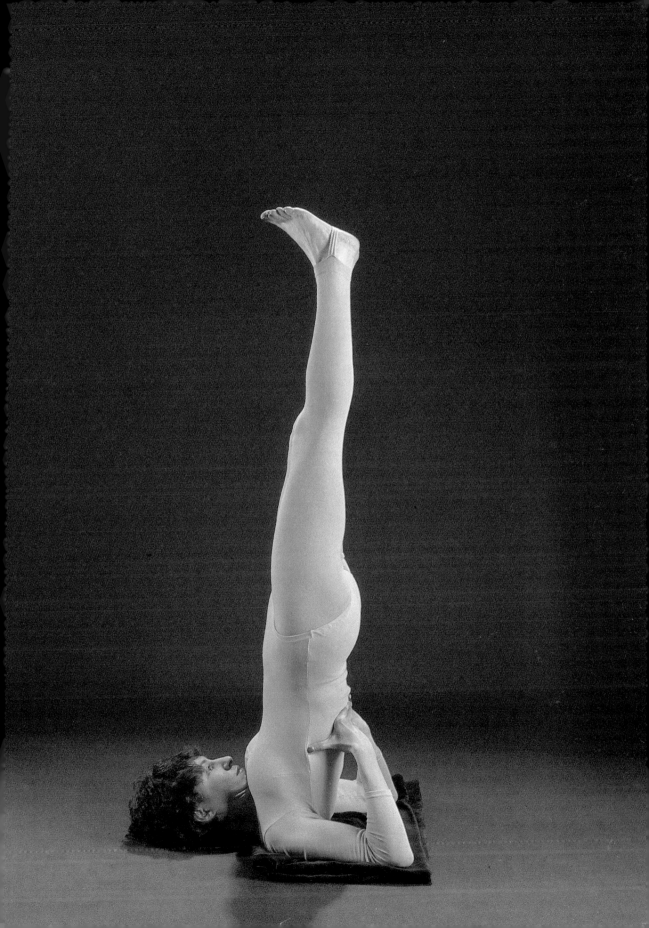

19 *THE FIRM POSE* Virasana

What it does:
Increases suppleness of the legs and helps cure leg pain, rheumatic joints and sciatica.

The lying back position stretches the abdominal organs and pelvic region.

Increases flexibility of the lower spine.

Points to remember:
Have a soft support under your legs.

Relax the buttocks down to the floor between the feet.

Relax back very gently.

Try to have the back flat against the floor in the final position, without hollowing the small of the back.

1 Sit back between your heels, gently persuading the buttocks to come to the floor between the feet. If that's impossible place a cushion underneath the buttocks.

2 As far as possible, the top of the feet should be on the floor, soles and heels facing directly upwards.

3 When buttocks have reached the floor, slide the hands back, fingers facing forwards, and allow the arms to support you in leaning back, stretching the front thighs.

4 Hold feet and come back gently and slowly on to one elbow then the other.

Final position: Lie back between the heels with your back on the floor, and relax! Stay for 10 seconds.

Come out: By carefully raising yourself on one elbow, then coming to the sitting position. Ease each leg out carefully, give it a gentle massage and shake it up and down to re-charge the circulation.

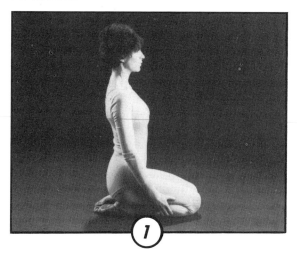

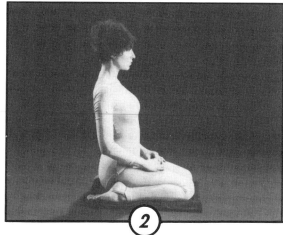

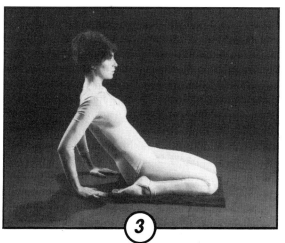

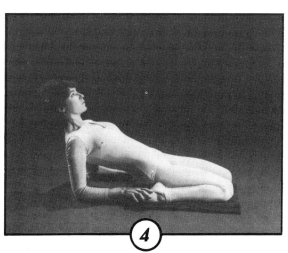

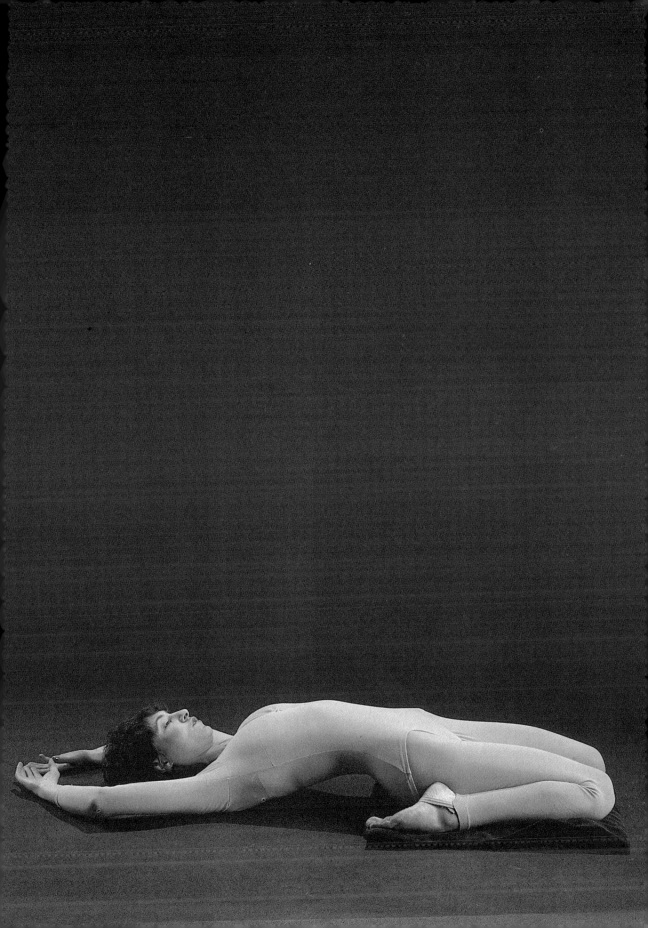

20 SPINAL TWIST 1 *Bharadvajasana*

What it does:
Helps make the spine supple.
Can help cure arthritic conditions.

Points to remember:
Try to keep the body firm, upright and balanced.
Open the chest as you move.
Do not strain the neck or eyes.
Try to keep both buttocks on the floor; if
    impossible, sit with a cushion under the raised
    side.

1   Sit with knees bent, and feet out to the left.
Place left hand on the right knee and the right
hand balancing the body on the floor at the back.
Twist body gently.

Finished position: Right hand reaches round the
back to hold the left elbow, thus bringing the body
round and twisting the spine in a 'wringing out'
movement. Stay for 10 seconds.

Come out: By letting go of the elbow and gently
moving the body back to face the front. Repeat
with the legs out the other way, to the other side.

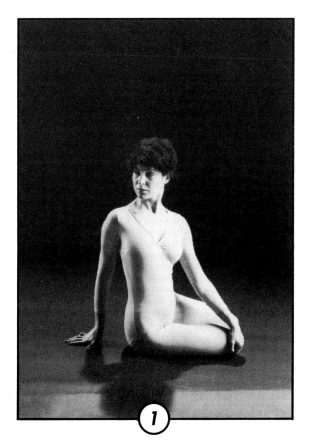

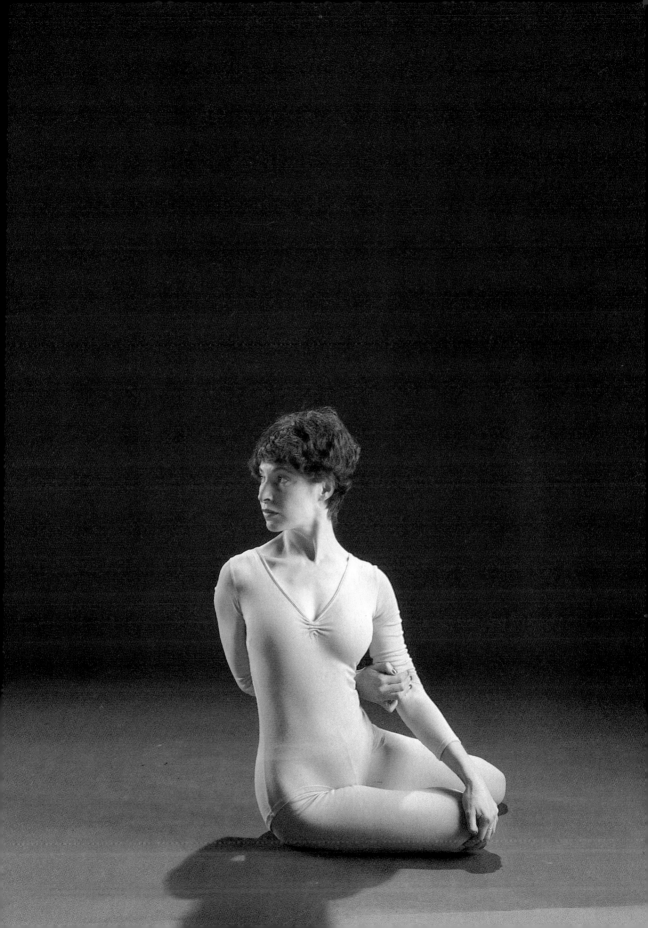

21 *SPINAL TWIST 2* *Ardha Matsyendrasana*

What it does:
Improves suppleness of the spine and hips.
Tones liver and spleen.
Relieves pain in shoulders and neck.
Activates intestines.

Points to remember:
Try to push the abdomen away from the thigh.
Sit well upright.
Expand chest.
Stretch out at the base of the spine.
Do not tense eyes, face or neck.

1 Place left heel against the right buttock. Place the right leg to the outside of the left knee. Clasp the right knee, and keep the back straight but not stiff, with both buttocks on the floor or a cushion placed to support them.

2 Move the right foot further back towards the left hip, and place the right hand on the floor behind the bottom for support. Begin to twist the body round to the right, moving the abdomen against the right thigh and keeping the back straight and chest even.

3 Move the left elbow to the outside of the right knee, twisting the body round further without hunching the shoulders.

Final position: Move the left arm under the right knee and interlock hands, 'locking' the body into the twisted position. Stay for 10 seconds.

Come out: By freeing the hands and turning the head then the torso to face the front. Uncurl the legs, stretch them out, shake them to relieve any stiffness, and repeat to the other side.

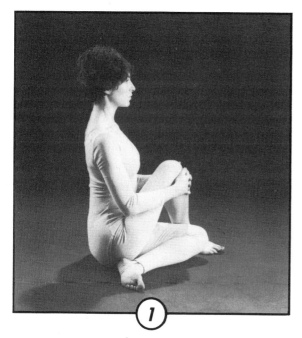

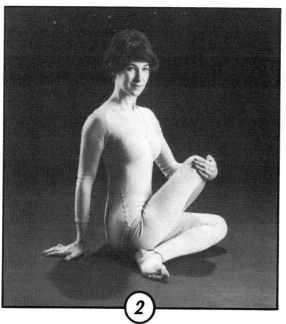

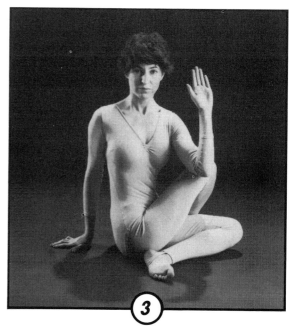

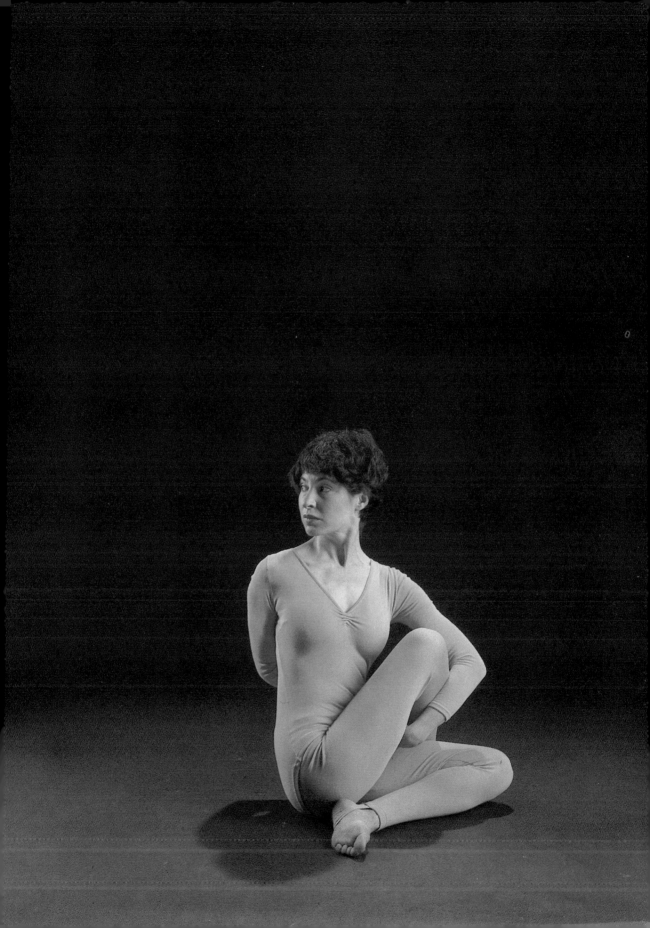

22 COW POSE Gomukhasana

What it does:
Relieves stiff shoulders.
Expands the chest.

Points to remember:
Stretch out the whole spine as you raise the arm.
Head should not bend forward or twist to the side.
Do not twist torso to one side.
Have a tie or scarf ready.

1 Kneel, sitting on the heels, keeping the back
straight and spine well stretched. Raise one arm,
attempting to get the elbow as far behind the
head as possible, the hand dropping behind the
neck.

2 Raise the other hand upwards behind the back,
keeping the elbow well in. You may clasp a tie
between both hands to draw them closer together.

Final position: Clasp the hands behind the back,
sitting well upright. Stay for 10 seconds.

Come out: By unclasping the hands and resting
them in the lap, easing off the shoulders and
making sure they are relaxed. Repeat to the other
side.

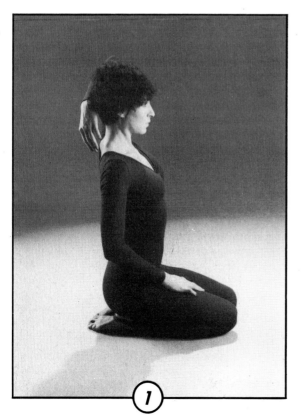

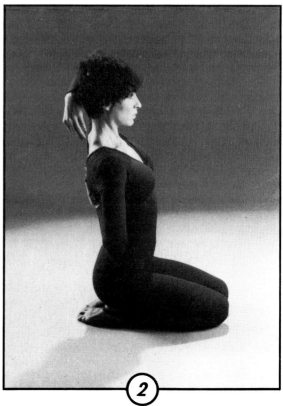

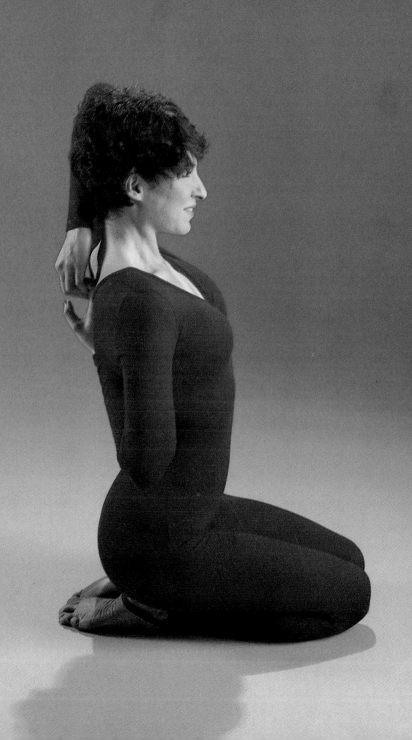

23 **BIRD** *Bhujapidasana*

What it does:
Strengthens hands and wrists.
Strengthens abdominal muscles.
Increases will-power.
Aids confidence and balance.

Points to remember:
Test the strength of the wrists by performing the
    first part of the posture a few times.
Concentrate on finding a point of balance.
Focus the eyes on an unmoving spot on the floor
    directly in front of you.

1 Kneel with palms outstretched on the floor in
front of you, and lean gently on the hands,
stretching the wrists and fingers.

2 Spread the fingers, balance in a squat on the
toes, and bend elbows slightly, pressing the knees
on to the upper arms just above the elbows. Find a
point where you can balance.

Final position: Tilt the body slightly forward, off the
toes, and balance with the arms taking the weight
of the body. Stay for 10 seconds.

Come out: By tipping back again on to the feet.
Shake out the wrists and arms to relax them.

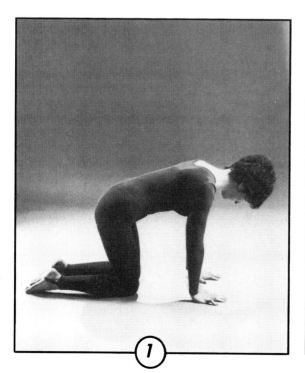

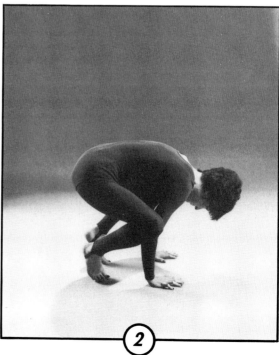

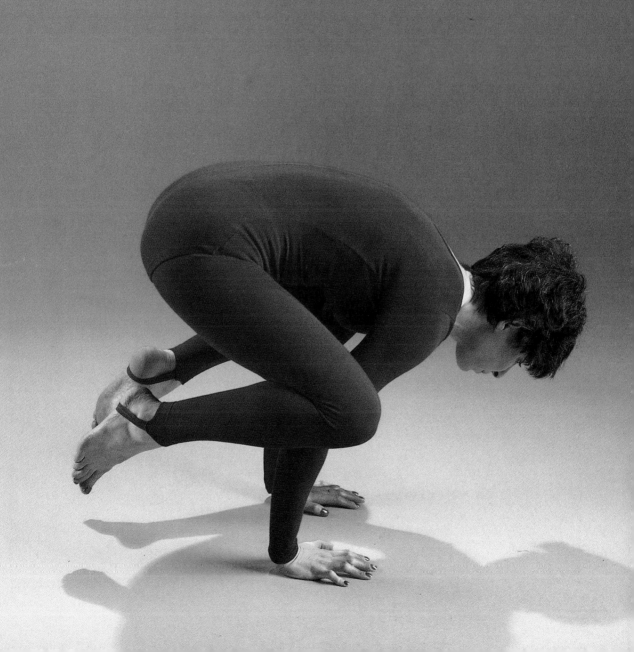

24 *COBBLER POSE* *Baddha Konasana*

What it does:
Helps cure urinary disorders.
Stimulates pelvis and abdomen.
Helps kidneys, prostate and bladder.
Helps menstrual flow.
Stimulates ovary function.
Helps prepare for childbirth.
Discourages varicose veins.

Points to remember:
Gently relax the inner thigh muscles to encourage
   knees to drop. Sit well up on the buttocks to
   keep back straight.

1   Sit with knees apart, feet together. Clasp feet
gently. Round the back and push elbows into the
inner corners of the knees, pushing them down
towards the floor.

2   Sit upright, allowing the knees to drop as far as
they can.

Final position: Knees pushed down to the floor,
back straight. Stay for 10 seconds, then alternate
three or four times with the bent back position.

Come out: By straightening the legs and shaking
out any tension.

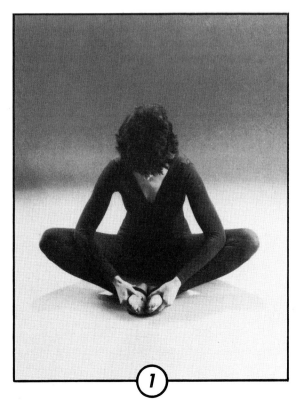

①

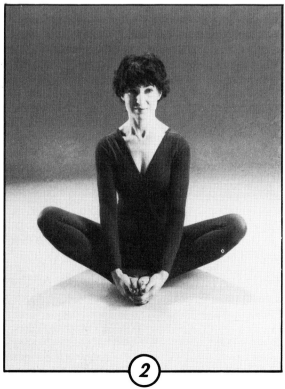

②

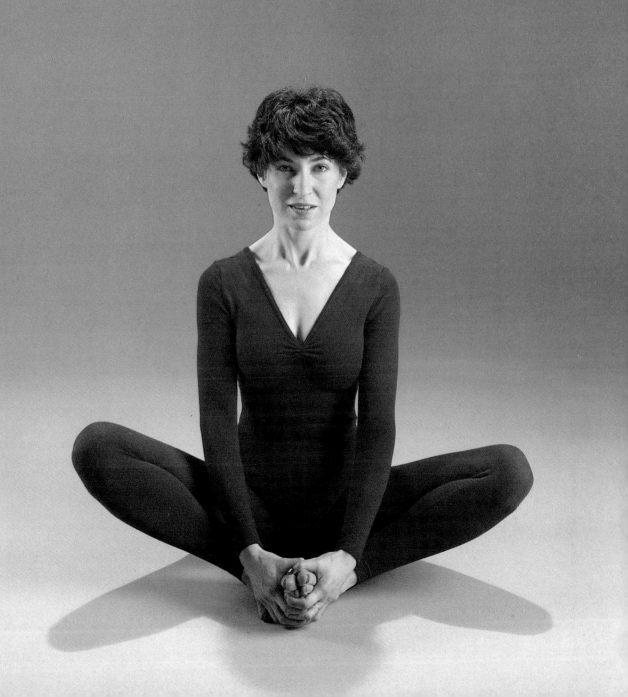

25 **LOTUS** Padmasana

What it does:
Creates a steady position, keeping the body still and the back erect.
Helps make knees and ankles supple.
Improves circulation in the lower back, toning spine and abdominal organs.

Points to remember:
Some people can do the lotus first time, some never achieve it — most people need several months of practice, so do not despair! Western limbs are very unused to this position. Constant persuasion and practice work wonders.

1 Sit well up on the buttocks with the right leg out straight, back straight, and the left foot on top of the right thigh, turning the foot so that the sole faces upwards. If this is impossible, just take the sole of the foot to the inside of the right thigh, and ease the left thigh muscle out with the hands. Keep both buttocks firmly on the ground — try not to tilt!

2 Gently ease the left knee down towards the floor, without tilting the body. Don't force anything — allow it to go when it's ready!

3 Bring the right leg up in front of the left shin.

4 Ease the right foot under the left leg — this is the half-lotus position.

Final position: The right foot comes up on the left leg, in the 'locked' full-lotus position. Stay for as long as is comfortable!

Come out: By disengaging the legs, and straightening them in front of you, shaking them to relieve any tension. Then repeat to the other side.

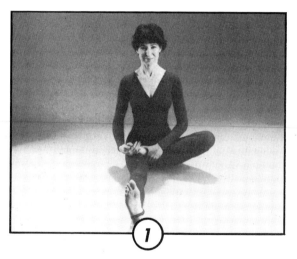

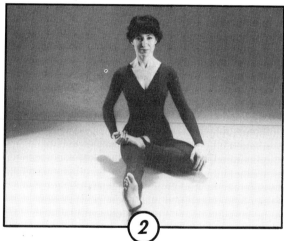

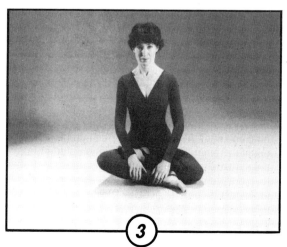

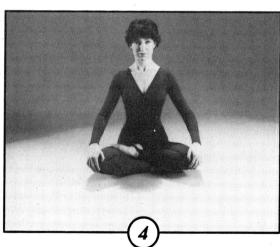

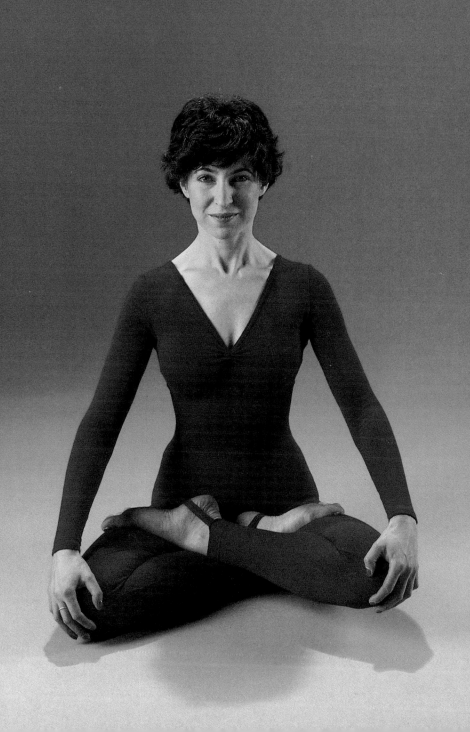

Chapter 8

YOGA RELAXATION

Relaxation is a state so basic for health, yet largely we neglect it until too late. Much is said nowadays about the stress of life, and while we know theoretically how detrimental it is to be constantly 'uptight', many of us get carried along almost without realizing how far we are from the true, deep relaxation we need.

Some tension is indeed useful — without it we would never get up in the morning or do any work. Pressure is what turns the adrenaline on, urging us to do better and go faster, to make that extra bit of effort and feel the resultant satisfaction. If such bursts of energy were followed by periods of rest, when body and mind become quiet and recuperated, all would be well. What happens usually, though, is that we become addicted to the state of tension. Outside pressures, increasingly hard to resist, spur us on, whether to perform better than the person in the next office, make more money, take more trips, get a better car, and so on. Our own internal pressure then responds to the clamour and complexity of modern life — we buy a freezer then use more energy scouring the supermarkets to stock it, insuring it against power cuts, and finding someone to service it when it goes wrong. Our inherent survival urge, which programmed in vigilance and energy, is nowadays stimulated hundreds of times a day, its original positive purpose turned negatively against our better interests. So we come to live in a state of constant 'arousal', straining at the leash no matter what our state of exhaustion.

This is fine when we want to achieve something really important. But what happens when we are unable to turn off the mechanism, (except artificially, by drink or drugs), and feel that we never, really, sit still and stop? We may carry on compulsively working, our brains churning with ideas, but with no constructive conclusion. We may become irritable, never able to show real empathy, love or affection. We may feel we're constantly putting on an 'act', with colleagues and even with friends. We become tired easily but sleep fitfully and wake unrested as when we went to bed. We may be aware of all these things, yet still be unable to counteract them, continuing with dest-ructive behaviour patterns we learn to live with.

Eventually the breakdown becomes physical. The effects of stress on physical degeneration are becoming well documented. Unrelieved pressure is a prime factor in hypertension, or high blood-pressure, and eventual heart attacks. According to individual weaknesses, tension's effects may be felt anywhere in the body. For some, it may come out in headaches, for others in such unsuspected areas as failing eyesight or skin disorders. Many authorities say almost every major disease man is prone to can be in some way attributed to stress, much of it deep-seated and long-held.

While for some time tranquillizers have been the answer for orthodox medicine, now the move is to self-help in the form of basic relaxation techniques and simple visualization exercises to reduce stress.

Here modern medicine is finally meeting ancient yoga. The practice of yoga has always included relaxation techniques. While the postures themselves were designed to keep the body strong and healthy, they also aimed at making it supple enough to sit in a totally relaxed way for many hours. Relaxation in yoga has a very specific purpose: to create stillness in body and mind so you are clear to concentrate, which in turn leads to the highly-esteemed state of meditation. Now of course a clear, calm mind and relaxed manner are being 're-discovered' and highly prized!

Although you may not want to meditate in depth, it is important to know how to relax at will. Many of us have our own favourite ways when the going gets tough. Watching TV, walking the dog, listening to music, taking up an absorbing hobby are some. In all these, though, you may not be as relaxed as you think. Have you ever had the sensation of a *really* good night's sleep — the kind where you wake knowing you haven't stirred since your eyes closed, where you feel weighed down on the bed like a stone, blissfully unable — and not wanting — to move? That's the kind of relaxation I mean, in that conscious waking moment where everything is *completely* undisturbed yet refreshed from your toenails to your soul!

With yoga techniques, that's the sort of experience you can create for yourself, whenever you want. Ideally, you can do a complete yoga relaxation at the end of your posture sequence. In fact ancient texts recommend that you relax after each posture, for the same amount of time you spend on that posture. Practically that's not usually possible, but it is sensible to lie and relax if you feel fatigued during your practice. You should have one brief (say, 5-minute) relaxation period in the middle of your sequence, and a longer period — 10 minutes if you can — at the end.

Otherwise, relaxation can be used any time. When you come home from work, mid-chores, whenever you feel the need. It is important to know you're not going to be disturbed — you won't relax completely if you're straining for the sound of the kids coming home or wondering what time the visitors will arrive. Make sure family and friends know this is *your* time — and that you'll be much more efficient, calm and able to deal happily with them afterwards!

It's hard to read instructions from a book and relax at the same time, so I suggest you either get someone to read them out to you as you relax (someone you feel unselfconscious with — and, preferably, with a soothing voice and calm manner!) or else, to read them yourself into a cassette recorder. Or you may prefer simply to read and practise them several times till you memorize them without difficulty and don't have to strain to remember what to do next!

When relaxing, do keep warm. Body temperature drops when you are keeping still and you'll immediately tense if you are cold. So wrap up with socks and woollies and a blanket if necessary.

You may place a thin cushion under your head, or a folded blanket, but do not use a feather pillow as it may make you drop off! The aim of full relaxation is not to send you to sleep — although don't worry if that's what happens. It is to enable you consciously to rest body and mind and to gain calm, still attention. Sleeping, your mind may remain active and you are not in charge: in relaxation, your own consciousness is directing the complete shedding of tension.

Here's what to do:
Lie flat on your back on the floor. Place the feet about 1½ ft apart from each other, and allow the toes to 'flop' outwards. Hands should be about a foot away from your sides, with the palms facing upwards. This may feel awkward at first, but don't be tempted to put the palms down. The palms-up position opens out and relaxes shoulders and upper back, and prevents any self-protection. The position is vulnerable and accepting.

Now mentally check your position — or ask a friend to do it for you. You should be symmetrically aligned — that is, if someone placed a broom handle down your middle there would be equal weight on both sides, its top would rest at your chin and both legs would be at identical angles from it.

Then check tension points. Is the small of your back rigidly curved leaving a large space between it and the floor? If so, gently release any tension here, without pushing it down — allow it to sink a few centimetres nearer the ground. If your shoulders feel like they're forming 'wings' round your face, do the same here — mentally place them on the floor and feel them descend, no matter how slightly. Chin is another danger point. Are you clenching your jaw for all you're worth? Noticing is enough to let it go.

All set now for the gradual, all-over falling away of tension. Start with your feet. The tips of your toes in fact. Feel relaxation in those toes. Feel lightness, draining away any tension, and let that sense of relaxation come up through the feet, all along the small bones and muscles as they lie there, perfectly relaxed. The relaxation continues, creeping its way up around the ankles — now the ankle bones, holding you over so many weary miles, can let go of their tensions too. Enjoy this new sensation in your feet.

Then allow the relaxation to come into the legs. It comes up from the ankles and unfolds into the calf muscles, it creeps into the shins. The whole lower part of each leg and foot is now heavy, and relaxed. The knees, too, become relaxed. Feel that relaxation working its way all round the knee caps, with their complex muscle structure, and round the back of the knees too. And then it comes up further, drawing its way — this warm, deep relaxation — into the thighs. All round the thighs it works now, front, sides and back, allowing you to experience their heaviness. Now legs and feet are wonderfully relaxed and heavy.

The relaxation comes up through the top of the thighs, it makes its way into the hips and all around the buttocks. If you feel any residual tension here that's hard to shake off, consciously re-tense the area making it even tighter, and then let go, completely, and relax. Now buttocks and legs lie heavily on the floor.

The relaxation comes up around your waist and deep into the abdominal muscles. Feel it here — there's no need to hold on, nothing to hold on to. Now you can let it all go, release all the long-held tension. What a relief it is, to allow yourself to let go. Now all the abdominal organs are relaxed and at rest. The waist expands slightly — no need to hold it in. Stomach too relaxes, just above the navel, and the area of the lower ribs too. Allow the ribs just to rest, their movements gentle and at peace.

Relaxation creeps all round the sides of the torso, and through the back — now your whole torso is gradually becoming heavier as it sheds tension, and you feel all the little knobbles of vertebrae in the spine, they too are comfortable and free from strain. All is warm and comfortable now that you're gradually letting go.

The relaxation comes further still, it concentrates on the shoulder area and all around the upper chest. The trunk is able to experience its full weight against the ground. Shoulders too are deliciously let go, there is nothing to hold on to now. The relaxation comes around the top of the shoulders, then makes it way down the arms. Upper arms, inner and outer, relax, and then the elbows, and then the forearms too, wrists and down into the hands, so often clenched and busy. Now you can leave them alone, rest them, and the fingers too, each one of their bones are at rest.

Relax your neck now, the back of it where it almost touches the floor, and the front — your throat and larynx. Chin and jaw are now let go; feel the cheeks relax and the tongue, resting gently behind the lower teeth. Lips part slightly as they too relax; let go of any tension in the nose and allow the relaxation to enter the eye sockets. Eyeballs feel as if they are sinking gently back into the head, so heavy are they, eyelids closed and at rest. The relaxation comes all around the temples, beside the eyes and into the forehead where any lines of tension are gently eased out.

Now feel the ears fall back, and the scalp itself is almost loose against the skull as it too relaxes. Now the whole body, without exception, is relaxed, each cell is at rest. Your whole body is sinking like a stone, it gradually feels heavier and heavier, like a big, leaden stone.

Now have an image of a warm sandy beach. No one else is on it, there is nothing but this big, heavy stone that is you. The sand is soft, warm, white gold. Grains shift gently as this stone sinks into it, settling into its warm, peaceful resting place. You are held by the soft sand, warmed by the sun. As you look up into the vast expanse of pale blue sky above, become aware of any thoughts that might be drifting through your mind at this moment — troubling, irritating, pleasing, it doesn't matter, don't try to categorize or judge them. As you become aware of a thought, see it written up in the sky. Now a passing cloud comes into view. It obscures the thought, drifts off taking it away. Now the sky is cloudless again, blue and pure. Should another thought come into consciousness, again, see it up above, way up away from the relaxed, heavy, weighted stone that is you resting in the soft sand. Another cloud comes, the thought is gone, you are less and less burdened, more and more free.

Now it is time to come back to life again. The images of sand and sky begin to fade. Bring your concentration back into your body, and especially into your breathing. Sense the stream of air coming in through the nostrils and into the lungs. Begin to deepen the breath, allow the ribs to move more fully, and the lungs to expand. Breathe to the bottom of the lungs, very slowly, gradually, gently. Take three of these breaths, then begin to feel your fingers, touch them together, move the hands. Then the feet come back to life, wriggle the toes, and the ankles.

Gradually begin to stretch. Lift the arms up over the head to touch the floor beyond, as if you are waking up in the morning. Keep the eyes closed, stretch all down one side of the body — right fingertips, right hand, side, leg and foot, relaxing the left side. Now stretch out the left side, relaxing the right. Now the left leg and right arm stretch (keeping everything else relaxed), then the right leg and left arm. Relax again for a few seconds. Place the palms of your hands gently over your eyes and open them, then when you feel ready, take the palms away and roll slightly to your left side to get up. Sit for a few seconds before getting up completely and carrying on with your relaxed, unstressful life!

Remember, life is full of pressures and sometimes we get so swept up in them it's hard to remember our own well-being. But whatever you do, you have the choice — to carry stress in your body and mind or to act from the fullness of your own harmony. To choose with conscious awareness is to be truly in charge.

Chapter 9

COMPOSING YOUR OWN SEQUENCE

The postures shown are classic yoga asanas. But no-one is expecting you to go straight into all twenty-five of them first time. They take working up to, and working into. The suggestions in the chart will help you to familiarize yourself with the postures gradually, at different stages of life.

People often wonder whether order of postures matters. It *is* important to get a correct sequence, although there are several different schools of thought on what is actually correct. Basically, the order depends very much on the idea of pose and counter-pose — that is, if you bend your back in one way, it makes sense to counteract that movement with a stretch in the opposite direction to even things out. As you become used to the postures, you will begin to feel for yourself how the sequence balances out.

This particular sequence is loosely based on the Iyengar system, which puts the standing poses first. These are more energetic and also give the whole body, in particular the legs and hip area, a good stretch, in preparation for the later postures. You will find that the following seated and lying down postures balance each other in stretching the body, and in particular the spine, in different directions. The Camel, for example, is an intense backward bending stretch, and is followed by bending forwards. Later, in the Cobra, the spine is again bent gently back; the lower spine is activated in the Locust and a very strong stretch is given to the whole back in the Bow posture. The Dog is then a strong counteraction to all these back bends.

Leg raising strengthens the body, in particular the abdominal muscles, in preparation for the Headstand and Shoulderstand, which need a firm, strong body more than balance alone. Spinal twists, as their name implies, flex the spine in different directions, and special attention is given to the shoulders, arms, wrists and hands in the Cow and Bird poses. Cobbler and Lotus positions work on often neglected areas of the thighs and hips. But at the same time as these specifics, the whole body is always involved in each yoga posture.

Here are some guidelines, then, to work out your own yoga programme, gradually mastering the complete series in your own time. Remember, there is no right and wrong for anyone. These are suggestions only. The basis of yoga is to feel your own way into the postures, using them for greater awareness of your own needs.

I suggest that everyone does the initial warm-up sequence (Chapter 4) as far as they are able. Take it as a gentle limbering, and if anything seems too strenuous, either leave it out or gradually work your way into it in a modified fashion.

The Cat posture can then be done by everyone.

The Salute to the Sun can be done if desired.

The postures should then be added in stages, as indicated. These stages are only guides. When you move on to include extra postures is entirely up to you. You do not have to reach the final position in order to continue to the next stage. You need only feel you have mastered the initial step(s) of the postures in Stage One. This will give you time to familiarize yourself with the postures and understand what you are doing, without trying to do too much at once.

Yoga is very much an individual progression, and how you move depends on what you've done before and how you're built. Some of you may find Stage One simple and go quickly on to the wider range of postures in Stage Two. Others will take longer. Sense how your own body is doing and what it wants. Going on to the next stage need not preclude your progress in the postures you are starting to master. Increase your proficiency in these as you add new ones to your schedule.

Small Children

Children are naturally flexible. You only have to watch them sucking their toes with the greatest of ease, or the natural way they fall, or hold their spines erect, to see how rigid most adults are in contrast! Usually the trouble starts when they begin school, and sit all day at badly-designed desks, later slouching over books and television.

Children should be encouraged from the earliest days to maintain their natural flexibility. They are usually intrigued by yoga postures, especially if they see adults doing them, but their concentration span is limited, so get them to do ones with interesting names, and make their sessions as much fun as possible, with plenty of challenge and encouragement.

Teenagers
Usually have lots of energy, but those school years and rapid spurts of growth encourage stiffness. It helps to maintain a regular programme.

Beginning Adults
Includes anyone past teenage years who is in reasonable health, but is unused to much exercise and does not consider themself to be particularly supple or in good shape. Get the feel of your Stage One sequence for a few weeks, then you should be able to progress with ease. Remember, you do not have to be perfectly adept before continuing to the next stage, but add in new postures when you feel reasonably confident of the step you have reached — then continue to work on these and the rest!

Fit Adults
Adults who do regular exercise and think they are strong and in good shape. Remember, though, that even when you are fit, you are not necessarily supple. Allow the muscles to stretch and relax as you do these postures, rather than aiming for the final position straight away. Yoga is a whole different game to competitive sport, so think of flexibility and ease as your prime motivation.

Over Sixties
It's really up to you to choose how far to go with your postures. Some of you may be fighting fit, others not so. Feel your way into the postures, see what's right for you. Stay at Stage One if it's tough — that much will still aid flexibility and delay degeneration. If you feel fine, go on and work up to the whole sequence.

Special conditions

Asthmatics
Concentrate on the breathing exercises in Chapter 5 and the postures as indicated.

Arthritis sufferers
Concentrate on the indicated postures, or as far as you can go towards them.

Obesity
Yoga can reduce overweight because it helps you become more aware of your body. The postures help balance the metabolism, too, particularly thyroid function which can influence weight gain. Take the postures gradually and concentrate on how you feel while moving and afterwards. Try to maintain a feeling of balance and allow your body to tell you when to eat rather than being ruled by appetite. Ask, am I really hungry? What do I really want just now? How is this going to affect my yoga postures? If you find you are just reaching for food from habit, or the desire for comfort — try doing a few yoga postures instead! The Salute to the Sun sequence is recommended daily.

High blood-pressure
While yoga cannot treat heart attacks, it is a known means of lowering blood-pressure and thus may avert emergencies. Comfortable yoga breathing exercises are recommended, plus the postures indicated and deep relaxation sessions. It is advisable to consult your doctor if you are considering starting yoga practice and suspect, or know, you have high blood-pressure. Never practice the headstand if you suffer from high blood-pressure.

Colds
These are natural cleansing processes, no matter how much publicity is given to quick 'cold cures' and treating them as if they're not meant to happen! Unless your body is telling you to rest completely, you should continue with your normal yoga programme. Particularly beneficial are the Forward Bend, Headstand (do just the first stages if you can't master it all) and Shoulderstand. Breathing exercises are helpful. Another useful yoga way of treating colds is the following: kneel on all fours. Breathe in deeply, then, on a strong outbreath, stick your tongue out at the same time as thrusting your neck forward so your head is sticking out as far as it will go. (It's preferable to do this in the privacy of your own room!) Sounds weird, but it does work. A kind of forcable eviction of the cold!

Stress, nervousness, mental problems
Increasingly common nowadays, but can be alleviated with regular yoga practice. Regularizing, harmonizing postures are indicated, with some that strengthen the nervous system. Regular practise of the breathing exercises will help too, especially alternate nostril breathing. Salute to the Sun sequence is particularly recommended.

Pregnancy
A special category which is not dealt with in this

book, because there are several excellent ones available which treat it with the detail it deserves. Although most of the postures can be done throughout pregnancy (so long as there are no complications and your doctor agrees), there are specific modifications as pregnancy progresses. You will need special exercises to strengthen your back and abdominal muscles, and the pelvic area, in preparation for the birth. You will also need to attend to your breathing and relaxation. The regular yoga sequence can help immeasurably in preparing the body to become fit and healthy before pregnancy, but I strongly recommend following the instructions from a specialized yoga and pregnancy book, in conjunction with a good teacher, once you become pregnant.

A Review of Your Complete Yoga Programme:

1 Warm-ups (Chapter 4)
Everybody should attempt these before anything else. They are essential to prepare your body for the postures, and need not take more than 10 minutes. Even children can go through them as a fun routine. Over-sixties should go carefully, not over-exerting themselves if they are unfit.

2 Yoga breathing (Chapter 5)
Everybody can attempt the simple yoga breath. Additional breathing exercises can be done if desired. Everybody can do the yoga breath plus movement. (End of Chapter 4).

3 The Cat sequence
Attempted by everybody.

4 Salute to the Sun sequence (if desired)
Particularly useful for teenagers, adults, in cases of obesity and stress. And for anybody who has no time for any other yoga postures, as a start to the day.

5 The Yoga postures
The complete twenty-five-posture sequence is gradually worked up to by some groups, as indicated in the chart. Others only do part of the sequence. Gradually familiarize yourself with the postures in each Stage, taking them one step at a time, according to the numbered pictures, and becoming strong and confident at each step as a position in itself.

6 Yoga relaxation
Everybody should relax at the end of the yoga session (Chapter 8).

YOGA POSTURE CHECKLISTS

	ASTHMATICS	ARTHRITIS	OBESITY Stages				HIGH BLOOD-PRESSURE	COLDS	STRESS, NERVOUSNESS, MENTAL PROBLEMS Stages		
			1	2	3	4			1	2	3
Tree		✓									✓
Wide leg stretch											
Triangle		✓								✓	✓
Warrior 1											✓
Warrior 2											
Sideways leg stretch											
Head to Knee											
Gate											
Camel	✓										
Forward Bend				✓	✓		✓	✓	✓	✓	✓
Forward Bend over one leg											
Cobra	✓		✓	✓	✓					✓	✓
Locust			✓	✓	✓						
Bow				✓	✓						✓
Dog	✓									✓	✓
Leg raising	✓		✓	✓	✓						
Headstand								✓			
Shoulderstand	✓			✓				✓			✓
Firm pose	✓						✓				✓
Spinal twist 1		✓			✓						✓
Spinal twist 2					✓						
Cow		✓									
Bird											
Cobbler							✓				
Lotus		✓					✓				

	CHILDREN	TEENAGERS			
		Stage 1	Stage 2	Stage 3	Stage 4
Tree	✓		✓	✓	✓
Wide leg stretch	✓			✓	✓
Triangle	✓	✓	✓	✓	✓
Warrior 1		✓	✓	✓	✓
Warrior 2			✓	✓	✓
Sideways leg stretch				✓	✓
Head to Knee			✓	✓	✓
Gate		✓	✓	✓	✓
Camel		✓	✓	✓	✓
Forward Bend	✓	✓	✓	✓	✓
Forward Bend over one leg			✓	✓	✓
Cobra	✓	✓	✓	✓	✓
Locust		✓	✓	✓	✓
Bow					✓
Dog	✓	✓	✓	✓	✓
Leg raising		✓	✓	✓	✓
Headstand					✓
Shoulderstand		✓	✓	✓	✓
Firm pose	✓	✓	✓	✓	✓
Spinal twist 1	✓	✓	✓	✓	✓
Spinal twist 2			✓	✓	✓
Cow	✓	✓	✓		✓
Bird			✓	✓	✓
Cobbler	✓	✓	✓	✓	✓
Lotus		✓	✓	✓	✓

	BEGINNING ADULTS				FIT ADULTS			OVER SIXTIES		
	Stage 1	Stage 2	Stage 3	Stage 4	Stage 1	Stage 2	Stage 3	Stage 1	Stage 2	Stage 3
Tree	✓	✓	✓	✓	✓	✓	✓			✓
Wide leg stretch		✓	✓	✓	✓	✓	✓		✓	✓
Triangle	✓	✓	✓	✓	✓	✓	✓	✓	✓	✓
Warrior 1		✓	✓	✓	✓	✓	✓			
Warrior 2				✓		✓	✓			
Sideways leg stretch			✓	✓		✓	✓			
Head to Knee			✓	✓	✓	✓	✓			✓
Gate	✓	✓	✓	✓	✓	✓	✓		✓	✓
Camel			✓	✓		✓	✓			
Forward Bend	✓	✓	✓	✓	✓	✓	✓	✓	✓	✓
Forward Bend over one leg		✓	✓	✓		✓	✓			✓
Cobra	✓	✓	✓	✓	✓	✓	✓	✓	✓	✓
Locust		✓	✓	✓	✓	✓	✓			✓
Bow			✓	✓		✓	✓			
Dog	✓	✓	✓	✓	✓	✓	✓		✓	✓
Leg raising	✓	✓	✓	✓	✓	✓	✓		✓	✓
Headstand				✓			✓			
Shoulderstand		✓	✓	✓	✓	✓	✓			✓
Firm pose			✓	✓	✓	✓	✓		✓	✓
Spinal twist 1	✓	✓	✓	✓	✓	✓	✓	✓	✓	✓
Spinal twist 2			✓	✓		✓	✓			✓
Cow	✓	✓	✓	✓	✓	✓	✓		✓	✓
Bird			✓	✓	✓	✓	✓			
Cobbler	✓	✓	✓	✓	✓	✓	✓	✓	✓	✓
Lotus		✓	✓	✓	✓	✓	✓			✓

INDEX